SEVEN KEYS TO REJUVENATION

Take Radical Steps to Look and Feel Ten Years Younger

Laith Doory

TABLE OF CONTENTS

INTRODUCTION

My aim for this book is to enlighten the reader with regards to the broad subjects of health, diet and fitness in a succinct and well thought-out manner without resorting to too much technical jargon or too many personal narratives. The key to health is a good diet, and any good diet should take on board the principals of the many well-known diets and refine them. Few things of any merit are created overnight.

Being in my fifties with a huge appetite and a propensity to put on weight, I have tried over the years almost every diet under the sun: the Hay diet, the Atkins diet, the ketogenic diet, alternate-day fasting, calorie counting; you name it. However, most people think I am still in my thirties, so I must be doing something right.

The regimen set out in this book should go a long way to helping you achieve what you thought was impossible without artificial help. Your own hormones cost nothing and do not come with a health warning. With this regimen, you should be able to optimize your natural potential by manipulating your own hormones with food combining and various supplements.

The regimen set out in this book is highly adaptable, there is no calorie counting, you can eat almost anything you want and you never have to go hungry, but you will need to be painstaking. Nothing in life is that easy.

Do not underestimate the latent power within you. Picture how you wish to look and know that it is attainable. If you have the key, you can open the door to the new you.

Disclaimer

Fasting apart, eating healthily or taking supplements can incur a heavy financial burden for some, but eating on a budget is not a part of the remit of this book. The purpose of this book is to enlighten, to put you on the right track and for you to make your own judgments as to what to consume, financial cost permitting.

In this information age, much of the information imparted in this book is readily available to anybody who would take the time to search it out, and I would actively encourage anybody who takes an interest in any particular supplement or subject to make further investigations before embarking upon any change in regimen. Withal anybody with health considerations should always consult a medical practitioner.

Chapter One

Key 1:
Alkalinize Your Diet for Better Health and Weight Loss

Our bodies naturally have a slightly alkaline PH. We have many mechanisms that try to maintain this normal PH level, but if the digestive system is constantly bombarded with acid-forming foods over many years, these mechanisms eventually break down.

Due to a modern diet bereft of fresh fruit and vegetables and often dependent on animal protein, wheat, sugar, processed foods, microwaved foods, carbonated drinks and alcoholic beverages, the body chemistry can tilt toward the acidic with dire consequences for your wellbeing. Acidosis is a condition characterized by an abnormally raised acidity that is highly detrimental to health.

Even if you do not suffer the ill effects of acidosis, long term, a diet high in acid-forming foods will make you more prone to weight gain, as this is one of the mechanisms by which the body tries to maintain a normal PH level. As a result, you will find it evermore difficult to lose surplus body fat, which the body uses to protect itself from excess acid. A high-protein diet consisting of mostly animal protein may give you a short-term weight loss, but long term the consequences can be disastrous.

The Symptoms of Acidosis Include:
• Acidosis creates an environment friendly to microorganisms such as bacteria, parasites, fungi and viral infections. One of the consequences of this is to upset the balance of your digestive system and can give rise to food intolerances, bloating and irritable bowl syndrome.

• It has an effect on the immune system, giving rise to autoimmune diseases and an increased susceptibility to allergens.

• A compromised immune system will make you more prone to infection: frequent colds, bronchitis, sinusitis and pneumonia.

• An overly acidic environment reduces the biological terrain's oxygen level and gives rise to low-energy levels and chronic fatigue.

• An increased bacterial level on the skin can give rise to acne.

• Bacteria, fungi and viruses can attach themselves to the inner walls of arteries and form a plaque that restricts the flow of blood. If this plaque build-up occurs within the coronary artery, it can give rise to heart disease, and if this happens in the brain it can lead to memory loss and ultimately to Alzheimer's dementia.

• Acidosis can undermine the skeletal system and can give rise to joint pains, arthritis and osteoporosis, as well as making teeth brittle and more prone to decay. Although other factors may contribute to the onset of such maladies, acidosis is arguably one of the main culprits.

• A slightly acidic body chemistry creates an environment in which cancer cells can multiply, where as a slightly alkaline body-chemistry will inhibit or even reverse the development of cancer.

Acid-Forming and Alkaline-Forming Foods

As a general rule of thumb, animal products, processed foods, microwaved foods, refined sugar, wheat products, rice and almost all alcoholic beverages can be considered acid forming. Though certain foods are more acid forming than others.

Unfortunately, these days many normally vegetarian livestock are fed animal feed containing animal protein and all manner of highly processed, GMO ingredients. Traditional grass-fed beef is higher in the essential fatty acid, omega 3, and lower in calories than beef fed with animal feed, and likely to be less acid forming. With regards to the consumption of meat, it is almost as important as to what the animals are fed as to the type of animal itself.

Ideally, meat dishes should be consumed no more than two or three times a week. For those that are concerned about losing muscle mass, one of the few sources of protein that is alkaline forming is whey protein.

Eliminating processed foods, microwaved foods and refined sugar should not be such a tall order. Nutritious acid-forming foods are good to consume as long as they are combed with alkaline-forming foods.

Fermented foods, cold-pressed oils and fresh fruit and vegetables are on the whole alkaline forming. Though citrus fruits are acidic, the majority are alkaline forming once digested, and it is this that is important to your body chemistry. Cider vinegar, unlike most other vinegars, is also alkaline-forming when digested.

Acid and Alkaline-Forming Foods in Detail:

• Fermented vegetables, such as sauerkraut, are highly alkaline forming if not pasteurized in which case they are mildly alkaline forming.

• Salad vegetables are highly alkaline forming.

• Almost all fresh or frozen vegetables are highly alkaline forming if not overcooked.

• Green beans, soybeans and white beans are alkaline forming.

• Corn, winter squash and olives (which are usually processed in some way) are slightly acid forming.

• Most other beans and legumes are slightly acid forming.

• Most pickled vegetables are highly acid forming unless home-pickled in cider vinegar.

• Canned and highly processed vegetables are acid forming.

• Microwaved vegetables are highly acid forming and best avoided.

• Figs, lemons, limes, cherries (sour), banana (ripe), avocado, tomato and watermelon are highly alkaline forming.

• Other fresh fruits are mildly alkaline forming or neutral.

• Blueberries, raspberries, cranberries, pineapple and pomegranate are mildly acid forming.

• Dried fruit tend to be mildly alkaline forming.

• Canned fruit are slightly acid forming.

• Potatoes (especially with skins), cassava, lentils and wild rice are mildly alkaline forming.

• Rice, pasta, couscous and bread are mildly acid forming.

• Aged cheese (blue or hard), soft cheese made with unpasteurized milk, goat's cheese, soy cheese and ewe's cheese are alkaline forming.

• Soft cheese made with pasteurized milk is mildly acid forming.

• Processed cheese is acid forming and best avoided.

• Soured milk, buttermilk, whey, live yoghurt (whole, unpasteurized), soymilk, goat milk and almond milk are all alkaline forming.

• Whey protein is mildly alkaline forming.

• Raw, unpasteurized cow's milk, fresh cream and fresh unsalted butter are neutral.

• Otherwise, most pasteurized and low-fat dairy products should be considered slightly acid forming.

• Margarine is acid forming and best avoided.

• Spelt, buckwheat, amaranth, quinoa and almond flour are alkaline forming.

• Wheat flour, oats and rye are slightly acid forming.

• Extra virgin olive oil (raw) and coconut oil (raw) are slightly alkaline forming.

• Regular heat-extracted olive oil and most other types of oil are either neutral or slightly acid forming.

• Any vegetable oil used in frying becomes highly acid forming, apart from coconut oil.

• Raw honey, raw sugar, unprocessed maple syrup and stevia are mildly alkaline forming.

• Refined sugar, fructose, pasteurized honey, processed maple syrup and artificial sweeteners are mildly acid forming.

• Homemade mayonnaise (with extra virgin olive oil) is slightly alkaline forming.

• Commercial mayonnaise and Ketchup are acid forming.

• Almonds and chestnuts are alkaline forming.

• Most other nuts are acid forming.

• Tofu (fermented) is alkaline forming.

• Textured soya protein is acid forming.

• Lemon and lime water are highly alkaline forming.

• Freshly squeezed orange juice is highly alkaline forming.

• Most other freshly squeezed fruit juices are alkaline forming or neutral.

• Sparkling water, all processed fruit drinks, fruit squashes and commercial sodas are acid forming.

• Herb teas and green tea are mildly alkaline forming.

• Regular tea, coffee and drinking chocolate are acid forming.

• Cider is the only alcoholic beverage that is alkaline forming.

• Wine is mildly acid forming.

• Liquors and bear are highly acid forming.

• Apple cider vinegar is alkaline forming.

• Most other vinegars are acid forming.

• Sea salt is alkaline forming.

• Table salt is acid forming.

• Raw fermented/cured meat, such as bresaola, can be considered neutral or mildly alkaline forming.

• Liver, organ meats and raw fish (sushi and smoked salmon) are mildly acid forming.

• Eggs, fish, chicken and duck are acid forming.

• Beef, veal, pork, tinned fish, processed sliced meats and sausages are highly acid forming.

• Any meat becomes even more acid forming if over-cooked or fried.

Microwaved Foods

Note that all microwaved foods are acid forming and best avoided. There is much scientific evidence to suggest that microwaving gives rise to a degradation in food that decreases the bioavailability of vitamins, as well as making the food carcinogenic ('Health Effects of Microwave Radiation,' by Dr. Lita Lee).

Alkalizing Supplements

Arguably the easiest way to help alkalinize your body chemistry is to breath heavily or hyperventilate, as this expels carbon dioxide, which is acidic. For those who are unable to improve their diet with enough fresh fruit and vegetables or wish to quickly reverse the harmful effects of acidosis, the following alkalizing supplements may help:

• The simplest way to alkalinize the body chemistry is to supplement with magnesium and calcium in recommended doses. Most people, however, already have plenty of calcium in their diet and supplementation with just magnesium should suffice.

• Citrulline malate has an alkalinizing effect on the body by boosting the body's natural bicarbonate level.

• HMB helps prevent metabolic acidosis, as well as many other health benefits.

• One of the few food supplements to have a strong alkalizing effect on the body is aloe vera, which can be consumed as a juice, but be careful not to buy a product that is highly processed or heat-treated.

• Bicarbonate of soda, which is a chemical used in many antacid preparations and in baking, has a powerful alkalizing effect on the body, but do not consume with food, as it neutralizes stomach acid. Always take antacid with a magnesium supplement as antacid depletes magnesium. Large doses of antacid can prove fatal.

Preparing Bicarbonate of Soda to Drink
Take a large beaker and add half a flat teaspoon of bicarbonate of soda to two to three tablespoons of cider vinegar. The cider vinegar also has an alkalinizing effect on the body but should neutralize some of the harmful effect caused by too much antacid in the stomach. Leave to froth, then top up with water. The taste of the vinegar should be completely neutralized.

This admixture is best taken on an empty stomach before retiring to bed, as the bicarbonate of soda can still neutralize stomach acid even if taken with cider vinegar. If food is not broken down by adequate stomach acid, it can ferment in the gut and give rise to all manner of complications.

An antacid should only ever be consumed with caution and is not recommended for long periods of time or as a substitute to healthy eating. Always take with a magnesium supplement to offset magnesium depletion. Do not take an antacid at the same time as any medication.

Chapter Two

Key 2:
Detoxify for Better Health
and Weight Loss

Modernity has brought about an exposure to toxins on a scale never before seen in human history from the air we breathe, prescription drugs, over-the-counter drugs, recreational drugs, anabolic steroids and notwithstanding many of today's processed and adulterated foods, many of which should come with a health warning. The body protects itself from these toxins by diluting them and storing them in water and fat. There are probably enough toxins stored in a typical middle-aged person's fat to kill him several times over.

When body fat is burned as energy, toxins that are stored in this fat reenter the bloodstream to be dealt with by the liver. This process is accelerated during an intense weight-loss regimen. Thus purging oneself of excess body fat will also have the dire consequence of releasing stored toxins.

If the liver is overloaded with toxins, it can give rise to rashes, headaches, nervous irritability, muscle aches, tiredness and a general feeling of nausea. If drug residues reenter the bloodstream, the likely result is a bewildering set of symptoms. Try to avoid remedying these symptoms with further drug taking, otherwise more toxins are simply put back into the body to replace the old ones.

In extreme cases a toxic overload can lead to a debilitating disease, such as multiple sclerosis, or premature mortality. Furthermore, any radical change in diet, such as the elimination of sugar, is likely to produce withdrawal symptoms that are likely to take time to remedy themselves.

Therefore if you are planning a fat-loss regimen, it is always advisable to begin this with a program of detoxification to help the liver cope with an increased toxic load. Apart from eliminating unwanted side effects, a program of detoxification should also help you speed up the process of losing stubborn surplus fat.

The Benefits of Detoxification:
• The mental benefits include increased mental clarity and heightened alertness, an increase in energy levels and better mood for those suffering from mild depression.

• Detoxification should make dieting easier.

• It will improve digestion by helping the liver function more effectively.

• It will lessen food intolerances that can lead to IBS or bloating.

• Chemical sensitivities and allergies are improved.

Mechanisms for Dealing with Toxins
Detoxification is a means of cleansing the body of poisons that are deleterious to every aspect of the body's efficacy. Though the body has its own mechanisms for handling toxins, these mechanisms simply cannot cope with the toxic load modern living places upon the human organism.

The liver is the primary organ for dealing with toxins. Glutathione, which is synthesized in the liver, is a powerful antioxidant that helps neutralize toxins and plays a key role in liver function.

Glutathione recycles other antioxidants such as vitamin E and vitamin C, which work synergistically. A diet high in antioxidants can therefore bolster liver function and help with detoxification.

Gallstones

The remnants of toxins processed by the liver can form gallstones. A gallstone can come in various sizes and can start out the size of a grain of sand and grow to the size of a golf ball. Most are expelled naturally whilst still small, but many may remain in the gallbladder and continue to grow. The accumulation of gallstones can hinder liver function, and very large stones may require surgery.

One of the few methods of helping to dislodge small gallstones is with the use of a caffeine enema. The caffeine dilates the bile ducts and helps the liver to release the body's accumulated toxins. A caffeine enema also stimulates the production of glutathione by up to 7 times. Coffee enemas, popularized by the Gerson Institute, have been used successfully to treat cancer.

Caffeine Enema

A caffeine enema requires little preparation and can be completed in less than half an hour. The caffeine enema has been popularized with the use of coffee, though arguably anhydrous caffeine is much cheaper and purer, given that coffee contains many toxins.

Use a two-quart enema bag, available from any drug store or ordered online. Though pure, filtered water is recommended, regular drinking water should suffice. Follow the instructions that come with the enema bag.

Add up to 400 mg of anhydrous caffeine to one and a half cups of warm water. A typical cup of coffee contains only 100 mg of caffeine, so be careful not to overdose. Do not underestimate the dangers associated with anhydrous caffeine.

A teaspoon of Epsom salt may also added to the water or used in a preliminary enema. Large amounts of Epsom salt can cause hypermagnesemia and prove fatal. Do not exceed one teaspoon.

Lie down on your right side and try to retain the caffeine enema for between 12 and 15 minutes. Do not force yourself to retain the enema if you find it too uncomfortable.

Bile has a strong, distinctive smell, and your stools should have a bile-like smell accordingly. If you start getting any other curious symptoms from doing a caffeine enema, you may be reabsorbing toxins through the GI tract.

To prevent this, take a toxin binder, such as activated charcoal, the night before on an empty stomach. You may also follow up the caffeine enema with a pure water enema to ensure that the bowel is evacuated of any remaining toxins and fecal matter.

You may use a caffeine enema daily for several weeks. Because regular enemas can cause potassium depletion, a teaspoon of potassium bitartrate (cream of tartar) may be added to your drinking water to compensate.

Epsom Salt and H2O2 Bath

Any hot bath will help eliminate toxins by drawing them to the skin's surface to be expelled. To enhance this process, you can add to your bath a cup of Epsom salt.

Soak in the bath until it is tepid. The Epsom salt is absorbed through the skin and helps draw toxins out of the body; it also promotes circulation, stimulates lymphatic drainage, relaxes aching muscles, neutralizes odors and softens and exfoliates the skin.

To boost the immune system, you may also wish to add food-grade hydrogen peroxide (H2O2) to the bath. Food-grade H2O2 does not contain the chemical additives of other hydrogen peroxide products.

The therapeutic water at Lourdes has a high level of naturally occurring H2O2. For those that cannot afford a trip to this French spa, a cup of 35% food-grade H2O2 can be added to a bath to soak in for about half an hour. This way, hydrogen peroxide is absorbed relatively safely through the skin.

H2O2 is a naturally occurring compound that is found in rainwater, fresh fruit, vegetables and colostrum, the first milk a mother produces, providing defense against infection. Honey and vitamin C are precursors to hydrogen peroxide when digested, giving them their curative powers. In the large intestine, acidophilus lactobacillus (found in live yoghurt) is another precursor to hydrogen peroxide, keeping at bay the harmful Candida yeast.

H2O2 is also known as oxygen water due to its composition of water (H2O) and an extra oxygen molecule. It is this extra oxygen molecule that is used by the body to oxidize and kill bacteria, viruses, fungi and even cancer cells. To maximize the effect of the hydrogen peroxide, supplement with up to 2000 mg of vitamin C prior to the bath.

Other Methods of Detoxifying:

• Alpha-lipoic acid is liver detoxifier and powerful antioxidant that recycles antioxidants such as vitamin C and glutathione. A dose of 50 to 500 mg a day is recommended. Best combined with biotin (vitamin B7) if this is not already contained in the formula. Never exceed a dose of 500 mg a day and do not take for any extended length of time.

• Apple juice and apple cider vinegar both help flush the liver of toxins.

• Astaxathin is a fat-soluble carotenoid known for its red pigment. It is by far the most powerful natural antioxidant. Doses can vary between 5 to 20 mg. As with any powerful antioxidant, it is not advisable to take for any extended length of time.

• Bentonite clay (food grade) absorbs toxins and heavy metals and rids the intestinal tract of Candida overgrowth.

• Vitamin C complex supplements of up to 5000 mg a day (in divided doses) can aid the liver in the production of glutathione. Vitamin C is also an antioxidant and precursor to hydrogen peroxide.

• Activated charcoal absorbs toxins from the gut, as well as intestinal gas. It is probably the most powerful detoxifier in that regard and can be a lifesaver for anybody who has been poisoned. Do not take activated charcoal with any medication or mineral supplements because it will be neutralized. Activated charcoal is best taken on an empty stomach.

• Burdock root detoxifies the blood and lymphatic system. As a diuretic, it also reduces sodium. It can be consumed as a food or in supplement form, up to 3 g three times per day.

• Chlorella is a type of fresh-water algae; it has countless health benefits, including protecting the body from toxins and heavy metals, such as lead and mercury.

• Dry skin brushing stimulates the skin to release toxins and rejuvenates the nervous system. Brush the skin with a soft brush before taking a shower or bath.

• Food grade diatomaceous earth can help flush the intestinal tract of toxins, heavy metals, parasites and Candida overgrowth.

• Vitamin E (natural D-alpha tocopherol) is a strong antioxidant. Doses can vary between 200 and 1000 iu.

• Herbs that can be used to detoxify the body include: dandelion root, mint and rosemary.

• High fiber foods, especially foods containing soluble fiber, bind with toxins so that they are naturally eliminated through the alimentary canal. Soluble fiber-rich foods include: oat bran, rye bread, whole-meal bread, brown rice, figs, prunes, apples, cassava, potatoes, vegetables, etc.

• Iodine supplementation can detoxify the body of heavy metals such as fluoride. Kelp, which can be taken in supplement form, is a natural source of iodine as well as many other minerals.

• Lemon/lime water consumed in large quantities can help flush the liver of toxins. Lemons and limes are also highly alkalinizing.

• L-taurine is a potent antioxidant noted for detoxifying the liver and improving liver function. The usual dose is 2000 mg up to 3 times per day.

• MSN (methylsulfonylmethane) is an organic sulfur compound found in many foods and is called a miracle supplement for its many health benefits. It works with vitamin C in the production of collagen and the elimination of toxins. The usual dose is 500 to 2000 mg up to 3 times per day.

• N-acetyl cysteine (NAC) is an amino acid and precursor to the powerful antioxidant glutathione. NAC is most noted for detoxifying the liver, as well as its many other remarkable rejuvenating properties. The usual dose is 200 to 1200 mg twice per day.

• Nattokinase is a digestive enzyme that detoxifies the lymphatic system, which works as your body's sewer system. For those with a sluggish lymphatic system, such enzymes are preferable to antioxidant supplements, which push more toxic residues into the lymphatic system, worsening the condition. Take 2000 to 4000 FU per day on an empty stomach.

• Raw, extra virgin olive oil consumed on a regular basis can help eliminate toxins.

• Psyllium husk is a soluble fiber that effectively absorbs toxins from the digestive tract. As a supplement, psyllium husk should be taken dissolved in water and allowed to swell up before consuming. If taken in pill form, always take with a large glass of water.

• Sarsaparilla is a South American herb known for its medicinal properties. It binds with toxins and purifies the blood. The usual dose is between 300 to 500 mg per day.

• Selenium is a powerful mineral antioxidant. The usual dose is 200 mcg per day.

• Triphala is an herbal remedy from Ayurveda medicine; it detoxifies and heals the bowl and is regarded as an overall tonic. Take 1 teaspoon per day in water on an empty stomach.

• Serrapeptase, like nattokinase, is a digestive enzyme that detoxifies the lymphatic system. Take 80,000 to 500,000 IU per day on an empty stomach.

• Turmeric is a natural liver detoxifier. It lowers fibrinogen levels and removes amyloyd plaque buildup in the brain, helping to prevent the development of Alzheimer's disease. Other detoxifying spices include: cayenne pepper, cinnamon and ginger.

• A sauna detoxifies the body by creating an artificial fever, purging toxins through sweating, as well as creating white blood cells to fight off viruses and bacteria. A sauna is also an excellent means of reducing sodium levels.

Chapter Three

Key 3:
Fasting for Rejuvenation
and HGH Production

A gas-guzzler consumes twice as much fuel as an econobox to take it the same distance. Therefore, if you transform a gas-guzzler into an econobox, you simply cannot go back to filling up the tank as you used to.

If you are very over-weight, past your mid-thirties and have never fasted or been on a serious diet, far from being predisposed to gaining weight, like a gas-guzzler, it is very likely that you are consuming approximately twice as many calories as you actually need. With so many calorific foods available in the modern diet, you are probably completely unaware as to how much you are actually consuming. It is probably a miracle of nature that you are not even heavier.

One of the reasons many people pile on even more weight after going on a diet is largely due to an increase in insulin sensitivity, which makes the body more efficient at utilizing calories and storing fat. This may sound like a bad thing for those intent on an easy route to losing weight, but a lifetime of over eating is aging, highly detrimental to overall health and will predispose you to diabetes.

An inability to put on weight might be seen as something desirable, but it is actually a sign of ill health. Somebody with type 1 diabetes will see a dramatic weight loss without dieting.

The good news is that healthier foods tend to be more filling and far less calorific than their junk-food counterparts, so at least in principle, you can dramatically cut your calorie intake without going hungry. In order to make any radical change in diet, you will need to look upon your relationship with food as something akin to a drug addiction. Just as any drug habit can be kicked with perseverance over time, so can you adapt to any kind of eating routine.

It could be argued that a person that has succumbed to anorexia has kicked the habit of eating altogether. Such a person finds eating physically painful. Of course, this is not something anybody should aspire to, but nevertheless this psychological illness illustrates the fact that there is little in your genetic makeup forcing you to eat large meals several times a day on a daily basis. Eating habits can be modified if you have the will, and once modified, it is something that can be of benefit to you for the rest of your life.

After any diet, once you have attained your desired weight, if you simply return to your old eating habits, you are doomed to failure. If you are serious about weight loss and keeping it off, you will need to face up to changing the way you eat for the rest of your life. Know your own body and your propensity for weight gain.

Fasting

Fasting and dietary laws are nothing new as far as most religions are concerned, though such endeavors were regarded as a matter of faith. However, the rigors of scientific research can now be applied to many of these ancient ideas, and fasting can be shown to have many remarkable benefits.

In the developed world, it is more often the norm to have meals three or four times a day, notwithstanding snacking between meals. Our distant ancestors, by contrast, often endured long periods of food scarcity. Our bodies have therefore evolved to adapt to eating patterns that most of us in the developed world no longer encounter. We have an ability to eat as much food as we can digest with a propensity to store body fat and with no stop button in readiness for a period of famine that never comes.

You might be aghast at the notion of a self-imposed period of food privation, but the human body is designed to cope with long stretches of starvation and runs far more efficiently on ketones from fats than on glucose from carbohydrates.

Moreover, a period of famine activates a powerful survival defense mechanism, not least a big increase in the production of growth hormone. This is something that can be utilized by athletes and bodybuilders.

Having said that, a fast can simply imply an abstinence of certain types of food, and it is in this sense of the word that fasting is employed for the purpose of maximizing HGH production. You will not be expected to go without food for any length of time.

Proteins and carbohydrates stimulate the production of insulin, which switches off the production of growth hormone. Conversely, growth hormone production is stimulated in the absence of insulin and will steadily increase for as long as insulin levels are kept subdued.

The Dry Fast

Autophagy, meaning *self-devouring*, is a natural process within the body whereby damaged cells, unwanted organisms and toxic residues are burnt as fuel. This has countless healing applications.

Dry fasting is believed to be three times more effective at inducing autophagy than water fasting and also far more effective at burning body fat. Supplements that can help with autophagy include: caffeine and acetyl L-carnitine.

For many, going without water is an even more daunting prospect than going without food, but certain beverages can help with autophagy. Coffee has been shown to induce autophagy in vivo. Caffeine is also a diuretic. Therefore the net effect of drinking any strong caffeinated beverage is to reduce the body's water stores and accelerate dehydration.

Apart from coffee, beverages such as matcha, black tea and green tea can also be used to induce autophagy. To maintain the effectiveness of caffeine, it is a good idea to occasionally cycle with decaffeinated beverages.

However, extended periods of dehydration can cause the body to store salt and to retain water as a survival mechanism.

Therefore it is not advisable to employ dry fasting too regularly. If you adopt intermittent fasting as a lifestyle, cycle water fasts with dry fasts on a weekly or two-weekly basis.

The Food-Insulin Index

A food with a low food-insulin index stimulates a minimum insulin response. Fats and oils do not stimulate an insulin response and salad vegetables produce a negligible insulin response. The good news is that many of the benefits of fasting can be achieved by cheating with such foods, which include: olive oil, coconut oil, MCT oil, butter, cream, soured cream, real mayonnaise, vinegar, pickles, lemons, limes, olives, salad vegetables etc.

Therefore, during a fast, you may wish to indulge in a salad made with salad vegetables, olives and olive-oil vinaigrette without feeling too guilty. You may also wish to conjure up a desert using as ingredients: cream, butter, coconut oil, coco powder and stevia, which is the only sweetener that does not produce an insulin response.

No matter how much fat is consumed, it will not be stored as body fat in the absence of insulin. You may crave carbohydrates, but you will not feel hungry.

During the fasting mode, coffee can be consumed as a beverage with cream, coconut oil or MCT oil and sweetened with stevia. MCT oil can be whisked and added to coffee as a creamer.

Coconut Oil

Coconut oil and its MCT oil derivatives are ideal to take during a fast because MCT oils quickly convert into energy and are utilized by the body in place of glucose. Coconut oil and MCT oils can therefore help maintain blood-sugar levels during a fast. MCT oils are also an appetite suppressant and will replenish energy levels and help with mental focus.

However, if you have never consumed these oils before, it is always best to add them incrementally to your diet lest you suffer an adverse reaction. For some people, coconut oil can be highly inflammatory and can congest the lymphatic system.

Improve Insulin Sensitivity

In a similar way that constant exposure to alcohol ultimately diminishes its potency, the body adapts to regular surges of insulin by desensitizing itself to it over time. As a result, the pancreas must increase insulin production to cope with the body's ever-increasing insulin insensitivity.

A person with insulin resistance can have a pancreas that pumps out up to seven times more insulin than the norm. Eventually the insulin resistance is too great for the pancreas to cope, bringing on the onset of type 2 diabetes.

In the absence of carbohydrate and protein in food, the body does not require insulin and the pancreas is rested. If the body is not exposed to insulin for a sufficiently long period of time, insulin sensitivity is improved as a result. Type 2 diabetes can therefore be cured simply by regular fasts on foods with a low food-insulin index.

Increase Growth Hormone Production

A 24-hour fast will increase HGH levels by approximately 2000% in men and 1300% in women, according to research at the Intermountain Medical Center Heart Institute. This increase in HGH peaks at the very end of the 24-hour fast. Positive effects of HGH include:

• An anabolic increase in muscle tissue.

• Muscles, tendons ligaments and bones are all strengthened.

• A change in metabolism that increases fat burning.

• Exercise produces an increased rate of fat burning for fuel.

• An improvement in immune function.

• Skin regeneration for a more youthful appearance.

Fasting to Gain Weight?

It may sound incredulous that you can gain weight by going long stretches without eating certain foods, but the massive increase in growth hormone production and increased insulin sensitivity can do exactly that. A bodybuilder can therefore utilize fasting as a means of gaining lean muscle.

Apart from the stimulation of growth hormone, increased insulin sensitivity will make insulin work more efficiently. Insulin is an even more powerful anabolic hormone than growth hormone.

However, increased insulin sensitivity will also make you more prone to storing body fat, as mentioned before, giving rise to the phenomenon of yoyo dieting. This can be avoided by managing insulin production, which is discussed in Chapter Four.

Alleviate Depression and Increase Energy

An HGH deficiency has been linked to psychological deterioration: increased irritability, depression, pain, tiredness and a decrease in energy levels. With increased HGH levels, regular fasts over time should lessen anxiety, help lift depression and give you a better night's sleep. You should feel more refreshed in the morning with more energy and a feeling of lightness.

Greater Mental Clarity

Fasting will initiate an improvement in mental clarity because the brain functions more efficiently on ketones from fats than on glucose from carbohydrates. If there are any carbohydrates in a meal, the body always utilizes the carbohydrates first before the fats with the exception of MCT oils and exogenous ketones.

Look Younger

A fast will give the digestive system a long needed break and divert energies to other things. Given that food digestion releases damaging free radicals into the system that cause aging, a fast reduces oxidative stress. Fasting also switches on mechanisms for cellular rejuvenation. Growth hormone affects the skin to improve its function and to make it appear more youthful.

Lose Addiction to Junk Food

Fasting will over time retune your relationship with food. It will re-sensitize your taste buds. When the body and palette are cleansed of toxins, you should gain the ability to fully appreciate the flavors of more wholesome foods. Processed foods with artificial flavors and additives will begin to leave a nasty taste in your mouth.

Heal Chronic Degenerative Diseases

Because fasting affects every aspect of the human body, it has a holistic effect on the body when it comes to healing. Where as conventional Western medicine can be relied upon for its invasive surgical techniques, its powerful antibiotics, antiviral treatments and array of drugs for dealing with the symptoms of illness, many of these drugs simply replace one set of symptoms for another broader set of symptoms or 'side effects' that are on balance more tolerable or less life-threatening.

Digesting food is very taxing on the body. Apart from the free radicals and the many toxic by-products produced from the digestion of food, it has been estimated that up to two thirds of the body's energy is directed into the digestive system after a heavy meal. A lack of appetite during an illness is a means by which the body diverts its resources from digesting food to fighting infection. During a fast, the body can utilize this energy in a similar way: for recuperation and to give the body a chance to eliminate toxins.

Because a fast will fire up your own physiological mechanisms for healing, almost any illness will see a significant improvement. Intermittent fasting is one of the most effective means of supporting tissue repair, reducing inflammation and boosting the immune system.

Of course there are no guarantees that a fast will resolve a particular ailment. Apart from type 2 diabetes, fasting should not be seen as a cure for any serious illness, but if you have any of the following ailments, you should certainly consider a regime of fasting as a means of improving overall health:

• anxiety/nervous tension

• atherosclerosis

• autoimmune diseases (allergies, arthritis, asthma, eczema, hay fever, psoriasis, rheumatoid arthritis, skin irritations and disorders)

• benign tumors

• chronic fatigue

• deterioration of the musculoskeletal system, osteoporosis, chronic back and joint pain

• gastrointestinal health (IBS, food intolerances, inflammatory bowel disease, leaky gut, ulcerative colitis, Crohn's disease)

• heart disease

• elevated cholesterol

• hyperactivity

• hypertension

• immunodeficiency

• insomnia

• lupus

• obesity

• premenstrual syndrome

• sinusitis

• sleep apnea (obstructive and central)

• substance abuse

• type 2 diabetes

• uterine fibroids

Supplements that Increase HGH:
• Citrulline malate, 4 to 8 grams per day

• L-arginine, 5 to 10 grams per day

• Vitamin B3 (niacin), up to 500 mg per day

• Melatonin for deep sleep, 5 mg before bed

L-arginine is best taken on an empty stomach for greater absorption. L-arginine HCL has greater bioavailability than pure L-arginine, though L-arginine HCL can deplete potassium in which case a potassium supplement is recommended to avoid water retention.

Alternatively, use citrulline malate, which is a precursor to arginine. Citrulline malate has greater bioavailability than L-arginine and is easier to absorb by the body, especially in older people. With either supplement, begin with a low dosage and gradually increase the dose over two weeks to adapt the digestive system.

Utilize the Fasting Mode with Your Workouts

Begin your fasting mode at least 4 hours before retiring to bed. Take L-arginine or citrulline malate before going to bed in a fasted state in order to increase HGH production during sleep. HGH levels will naturally increase for as long as you go without carbohydrate or protein.

Sleep will give you a further 8 hours or so of fasting. Deep sleep is important to HGH production, in which case supplementation with melatonin before retiring to bed may prove helpful.

The next morning, take another dose of either L-arginine or citrulline malate before going to the gym in a fasted state to maximize HGH production from the workout. Before heading to the gym, you may consume black coffee with added coconut oil or MCT oil, which will give you more energy. Oils and fats do not produce an insulin response and can be utilized to stave off hunger for the purpose of extending a fast.

Your subsequent fast should last between 13 and 14 hours in which HGH production is bolstered by the consummation of L-arginine or citrulline malate. At the end of the workout, you can break your fast with a protein shake.

A Regime of Regular 24-Hour Fasts

In addition to regular fasts incorporated into your workout regimen, you may wish to incorporate a single 24-hour fast into your weekly routine to maximize HGH production. You can modify these hours to suit your lifestyle, but always begin fasting at least 4 hours before retiring to bed. Unlike a starvation fast, you should be able to achieve a 24-hour fast with relative ease by consuming foods with a low food-insulin index.

Fasting is a lot easier than you might think, but if you have never tried a fast before of any kind, you are likely to find yourself lacking in willpower to put it mildly. For many, the idea of going without regular food for 24 hours is a daunting prospect, but over time, you will surprise yourself how easy it is.

If you set yourself a reasonable goal, which you then achieve, you can keep re-positioning the goalposts until you achieve your ultimate target. With regular practice, you will soon be able to go the long stretch by consuming foods with a very low food-insulin index.

Cautions

It should be stressed that any radical change in diet can have a detrimental effect on health and should only ever be embarked upon incrementally. Increased insulin sensitivity should stave off the onset of diabetes in old age, but if it comes about too rapidly, it can bring on the onset of reactive hypoglycemia. For this reason, fasting should only ever be introduced into a regimen slowly, especially if you are very overweight or over the age of 35.

If you suffer from hypoglycemia, it is not advisable to fast for any length of time. Anybody who suffers from this condition should consider a low-calorie, low-glycemic diet or a ketogenic diet. Eating regular, smaller meals should help, as well as supplementing with the following:

• Chromium, 1000 mcg twice per day

• Ceylon cinnamon, ½ teaspoon half an hour before each meal

• Apple cider vinegar, 2 tablespoons half an hour before each meal

• MCT oil

• Coconut oil

Supplementing with benfotiamine (fat-soluble vitamin B1) and niacin (vitamin B3) should counter some of the negative side effects of low-blood sugar.

Bad Breath

A 24-hour fast can give rise to bad breath, but this should soon alleviate itself over time. If you have persistent bad breath as a result of fasting, you may have a bacterial imbalance. If this is not caused by rotting teeth, foods and supplements that may help include:

- Vitamin C, 2000 mg up to 3 times per day

- Caprylic acid/MCT oil/coconut oil

- Live yoghurt (unsweetened)

- Cayenne pepper, ½ teaspoon per day

- Cranberry juice (sugar free)

- Extra virgin olive oil

- Chlorella, 1 to 2 tablespoons per day

- Probiotics

- Prebiotics (such as inulin)

- Activated charcoal, 1 to 2 tablespoons on an empty stomach

- 3% food-grade hydrogen peroxide, as a mouthwash

Chapter Four

Key 4:
Manage Insulin to Lose Weight and Gain Muscle

There are several factors that come into play when trying to measure weight loss, and a reading on a weighing machine can be very misleading. The notion that you can lose several pounds of fat in just one week is not possible given that the body can only burn so much body fat as fuel. Much of the weight loss is likely due to a loss of fluid and an emptying of the intestines of slow-moving fecal matter.

Weighing machines can therefore only ever give an approximate measurement as to how your diet is progressing and should only be used at most once a week. Fat calipers are more useful in measuring body fat.

Insulin

There is a lot more to dieting than calculating the ratio between calorie intake and calorie expenditure, and the manipulation of insulin production is arguably the key to any effective diet. Insulin manipulation is a useful tool for dieters, especially those who find it difficult to lose weight for whatever medical reason.

The main aim of a diet should be to lose body fat and to maintain or even increase muscle mass. In terms of volume, muscle weighs approximately twice as much as fat. A good diet can therefore have the net effect of increasing body weight.

Increased muscle mass speeds up the metabolism, which makes dieting a lot easier. Your body will burn more calories without having to monitor food intake or do any aerobic exercise. It is not unheard of for a bodybuilder to consume in the region of 5000 calories per day.

Growth hormone and testosterone are often cited as powerful anabolic hormones where as insulin is often called the fat-storage hormone, but insulin is actually by far the most powerful anabolic hormone under certain conditions. In fact, many professional bodybuilders are known to inject insulin for massive gains. However this is not a practice anybody should advocate because of its inherent dangers and long-term health problems, such as the onset of diabetes and the development of cataracts.

The following regimen employs some of the food-combining techniques of the Hay diet, but utilizes hormones to maximize muscle growth and reduce body fat. Four modes of eating are employed that alternate between a high-insulin mode, a medium-insulin mode, a low-insulin mode and a fasting mode, which was discussed in Chapter Three.

The high and medium-insulin modes can be utilized up to five days a week, and the low-insulin mode can be utilized on the remaining days. The fasting mode is simply a means of extending your fasting state every time you sleep for the purpose of boosting growth hormone.

Of course it is helpful on any diet to also do regular workouts at the gym, though this is not essential. Getting the most out of your workout program is discussed in Chapter Seven.

High-Insulin Mode

Unfortunately, the high-insulin mode does not involve the consummation of a huge amount of calories from carbohydrates but a targeted use of a relatively small amount of high-glycemic carbohydrates for the purpose of inducing an insulin spike. Whey protein can be blended into a shake with a high-glycemic carbohydrate, equating to a cup of fruit juice, such as: apple juice, orange juice, banana etc. Sugar can also be used for the purpose of inducing an insulin spike, but avoid consuming too many carbohydrates lest they be converted into fat.

In order to utilize insulin as an anabolic, it is imperative that fat consumption be at a minimum in any high-protein meal. The purpose of the insulin spike is to target the protein in your meal for muscle protein synthesis. If there is oil or fat in your meal, any insulin spike would cause this to be stored as body fat.

Do not use full-fat milk, coconut water, chocolate, or any food containing fat in your protein shake. The high-insulin mode makes use of low-fat protein sources, such as: whey protein, white fish, turkey, egg whites and tofu.

Whey Protein

Whey protein is an ideal source of protein for increasing muscle mass because it is a fast-release protein, virtually fat free and is not acid forming when digested. Whey protein has one of the highest protein contents of any food. 100 grams of whey protein provides about 80 grams of protein. This compares with 100 grams of turkey, which provides about 22 grams of protein.

MCT Oil

The only oil you can consume during the high and medium-insulin modes is MCT oil. Unlike any other fat or oil, MCT oil digests quickly like a carbohydrate and does not convert into body fat.

MCT oil is noted for improving brain function, stamina and stabilizing blood-glucose levels. Begin with no more than two teaspoons in any serving and increase your intake slowly over several weeks in order to adapt the digestive system.

Medium-Insulin Mode

Both high-insulin mode and medium-insulin mode can be utilized on the same day in different meals as long as they are adequately paced, preferably four hours apart. Where as the high-insulin mode is centered upon whey protein and the occasional inclusion of other low-fat protein sources, the medium-insulin mode is utilized for other types of slow-release proteins, such as: chicken, lean beef, tuna, salmon etc. Such protein sources can be consumed with any green vegetable and a small amount of low-glycemic carbohydrate, such as whole-meal bread. Avoid high-glycemic carbohydrates, such as: white bread, pasta, potatoes, sugar, etc.

Protein raises blood sugar and stimulates the production of insulin to a far lesser degree than carbohydrate. Compared to carbohydrates, most proteins lean more to stimulating insulin than raising blood sugar.

The release of glucose from protein, via gluconeogenesis, tends to lead to improved blood-sugar control and a reduced calorie intake due to a feeling of satiation. Protein also stimulates the fat-burning hormone, glucagon.

Apple Cider Vinegar

If you are a big eater, low-glycemic carbohydrates can still be converted into fat if consumed to excess, especially when combined with protein. To prevent this, consume 2 tablespoons of raw apple cider vinegar half an hour before each meal. This should be diluted with half a glass of water and drunk through a straw to prevent any damage to the enamel on your teeth. The apple cider vinegar helps to satiate hunger and to level off any insulin spike.

When Can You Eat French Fries?

Both carbohydrates and proteins produce an insulin response, and if they are combined in the same meal, the insulin response is compounded as an insulin spike. Combine this insulin spike with fat, such as that contained in French fries, and it is the surest way to pile on the pounds.

However, it is possible to diet and consume foods that are high in both fat and carbohydrates, as long as they are consumed in moderation and without any accompanying proteins. Wait at least 4 hours after any meal containing protein and consume 2 tablespoons of apple cider vinegar half an hour beforehand to lessen the effect of the insulin. So if you crave French fries or cookies or any food high in both fat and carbohydrates, if you follow this advice, you can indulge without worrying too much about gaining body fat.

Low-Insulin Mode

The low-insulin mode should help improve insulin sensitivity, stimulate the production of growth hormone and glucagon and supply the body with fatty nutrients essential to health. Use this mode to consume: eggs, olive oil, coconut oil, nuts, high-fat meats and good-quality cheeses, as well as fat-soluble supplements for better absorption.

Fat does not produce an insulin response. Fat is not stored as body fat in the absence of insulin, but burns as energy and blunts your appetite. In spite of a large proportion of fat in a meal, a very low insulin response should ensure that most of this fat is not stored as body fat.

The low-insulin mode is therefore centered upon the consumption of fat and oil whereby high-fat foods are consumed with little protein and the very minimum of carbohydrates from low-carbohydrate vegetables and salad vegetables.

Protein consumption should be below 30 grams per meal in order to minimize insulin production. Paradoxically, high-fat meats serve this mode better than leaner cuts, as high-fat meats have a lower insulin response.

The low-insulin mode does not need to be a low-calorie mode. Because the low-insulin mode quickly satiates your appetite, overall calorie consumption is likely to be reduced nevertheless.

It is feasible to switch from high or medium-insulin mode in the early hours to low-insulin mode later in the evening. However, do not start the day with a low-insulin mode and then switch to a high-insulin mode later on, as the fat you consumed earlier in the day is still being digested and any insulin spike will cause this fat to be stored as body fat. For a healthy person, an insulin spike usually lasts only a few hours, though the effects of an insulin spike can last up to 48 hours for people who suffer from insulin insensitivity.

However, do not use the low-insulin mode as an excuse to gorge yourself with a large amount of fat that your digestive system is ill equipped to handle. It is possible to go on a diet of bulletproof coffee and fried pork rinds and quickly lose a lot of body fat, but some people may suffer dire consequences. Therefore, it is always advisable to adapt the digestive system by making incremental changes over several weeks.

Note that all artificial sweeteners produce an insulin response apart from stevia. You may add stevia to your morning coffee, as well as cream or coconut oil.

Breaking The Rules

Though this regimen is designed so that you do not go hungry, if you do not follow the rules, you will need to compensate with a period of fasting. If you break the low-insulin mode with carbohydrates, cut down on your day's calorie intake accordingly in order to ensure a calorie deficit and consume apple cider vinegar for good measure. If all you eat all day is one beef-burger with a side order of fries, you will be in calorie deficit and still lose weight in spite of the insulin spike and high-fat content.

Eat Green Vegetables

Green vegetables are not only important for their dietary fiber, but are also useful to counter the acid-forming nature of most protein sources. Most green vegetables can be consumed in large amounts with the high, medium and low-insulin modes. Make green vegetable a dietary staple, but if you are not used to consuming large amounts of vegetables, you may have to increase your vegetable intake slowly over several weeks in order to adapt your digestive system and avoid bloating.

Chapter Five

Key 5:
Help the Adrenals to
Counter Stress

Unlike testosterone, growth hormone and insulin, which are anabolic hormones, cortisol is a steroidal hormone of the catabolic variety. Cortisol is released by the adrenal glands at times of physical exertion or mental stress, as well as first thing in the morning upon waking.

The functions of cortisol include:

• Fight or flight response that floods the body with glucose.

• Temporary increase in energy production.

• It inhibits insulin production.

• It increases the heart rate.

• It reduces protein syntheses.

• It breaks down muscle protein into glucose for energy.

• It balances blood sugar at times of stress.

• It governs inflammatory response.

Adrenal Fatigue

With today's hectic, stressful lifestyle, problems relating to the adrenals are all too common. Because cortisol is a catabolic hormone that predisposes you to losing muscle mass and putting on body fat, for any dieter, this is especially problematic.

There are many stressors that can bring about the release of cortisol from the adrenals, including: depression/anxiety, caffeine, systematic inflammation and excessive aerobic exercise and over training. Long-term elevated exposure to cortisol can give rise to adrenal fatigue and a variety ailments that are all too symptomatic of modern living.

Symptoms of Adrenal Fatigue:

• Anxiety, irritability, depression and bipolar disorder

• Autoimmune diseases such as eczema or arthritis

• Chronic fatigue syndrome

• Cravings for high-calorie foods

• Dark circles under the eyes

• Dependency on stimulants such as coffee

• Dizziness

• Elevated blood sugar

• Food allergies and intolerances

• Frequent urination

• Gastrointestinal problems and poor digestion

• Hypertension and cardiovascular disease

• Increased abdominal fat, weight gain and inability to lose weight

• Infertility

• Insomnia

• Insulin insensitivity

• Impaired immunity and susceptibility to colds

• Impaired memory and brain fog

- Lethargy during the day, but high energy levels in the evening

- Lower back pain

- Numbness in fingers and poor circulation

- Reduced glucose utilization

- Reduced growth hormone, testosterone and muscle mass

- Reduced libido

- Osteoporosis

- Thyroid disorders

- Type-2 diabetes

- Water retention

Managing Cortisol Levels

If stress is a problem, try to manage this as best you can by avoiding stressful situations. Limit caffeine intake and avoid any psychological stressors, including newspapers and TV news. Instead engage in relaxing pursuits and get adequate sleep.

If systematic inflammation is a problem, this can be helped by a change in diet. Avoid inflammatory foods such as: genetically modified foods, processed foods, high-glycemic foods, saturated fats, trans fats, microwaved foods, excessive animal protein, excessive alcohol and any food known to cause gastrointestinal irritation.

Though caffeine is an anti-inflammatory, caffeine raises cortisol levels and should not be overindulged. Anti-inflammatory drugs such as ibuprofen and aspirin may temporarily alleviate symptoms, but long-term use of these drugs can exacerbate systematic inflammation.

If you suffer from adrenal fatigue, maintaining blood-sugar levels is important to controlling cotisol. Eating first thing in the morning and directly after a workout are important, as well as regular consumption of protein or low-glycemic carbohydrates.

Though if you supplement adequately, you will still be able to utilize the low-insulin and fasting modes mentioned in Chapter Four.

Supplements for the Adrenals

The most powerful supplement for balancing the hormones is pregnenolone, which is a precursor hormone to all other steroid hormones. The recommended dose for pregnenolone is 100 mg up to twice per day. Otherwise there are a variety of supplements that can help the adrenals of which the most effective include:

• Ashwagandha, up to 2 g (powdered form) per day in divided doses.

• Vitamin B3, 500 mg per day.

• Vitamin B6 (pyridoxal 5-phosphate, the biologically active form), up to 100 mg per day.

• Vitamin C complex, up to 5 grams per day in divided doses.

• 5HTP, 200 to 400 mg per day.

• Licorice root, 450 mg twice a day.

• L-glutamine, up to 20 grams per day in divided doses.

• L-taurine, 2000 mg up to 3 times per day.

• Magnesium, up to 5 mg per pound in body weight.

• N-acetyl L-tyrosine, 500 mg up to twice a day.

Other supplements that may be helpful include: vitamin B complex, benfotiamine, CoQ10, vitamin E, holy basil, Omega 3, phosphatidyl serine, rhodiola rosea, RNA, ginseng and the minerals zinc and copper.

Exercise and Cortisol

Aerobic exercise is especially noted for increasing cortisol production, though this is offset to a degree by the release of endorphins. If you already suffer from adrenal fatigue, your symptoms are likely to be compounded.

Aerobic exercise may expend energy and burn body fat, but it will also burn muscle tissue due to the increase in cortisol. By contrast, weight-training gives rise to a relatively smaller cortisol response, and this is offset by a large increase in growth hormone.

Weight training is therefore the preferred option for those wishing to not only gain muscle mass but also to lose body fat. Keep weight-training sessions under an hour and allow adequate resting periods between training sessions to avoid over training.

Chapter Six

Key 6:
Reduce Fluid Retention to
Lose Weight

As a result of subcutaneous fluid, you may be carrying several kilos in weight in water that you assume to be body fat. You can test this on yourself: using the skin on your abdominal area, give it a pinch and pull it before letting go. If the flesh makes a significant quivering motion, you are likely to be carrying a large amount of subcutaneous fluid you assume to be fat.

Fluid retention is a condition that is a lot more common than most people realize and can be caused by a whole variety of reasons. Water retention is often spoken of in dismissive terms, but it is a condition that may take several months or even years to rectify and may have a serious underlying cause. This is not helped by a medical profession that does not have a reliable means of diagnosing this condition unless it is very pronounced.

In medical terms, ascites refers to fluid retention in the abdominal cavity and is most associated with heavy beer drinkers in the public imagination. Edema refers to water retention in any other part of the body, more often the lower legs.

If you believe you have any form of fluid retention, it is always advisable to consult with a medical practitioner in order to establish the underlying cause in case it is something serious. In severe cases of ascites, the fluid may have to be drained by a medical practitioner.

Stress, Salt and Aldosterone

The biggest causation factor when it comes to fluid retention is stress. When under stress, a hormone called aldosterone sends a message to the kidneys to retain salt, which in turn causes water retention. Potassium is also depleted. This is compounded by a modern diet high in sodium and low in potassium-rich fruits and vegetables.

Paradoxically enough, this is often further compounded by dehydration. When the body is slightly dehydrated, and most people do not drink the recommended 2 liters of water per day, the body tries to cling onto water reserves as a survival mechanism.

Furthermore, coffee acts not only as a diuretic, but also increases stress and aldosterone levels, which in turn depletes potassium and raises sodium. Coffee is noted for its ability to burn body fat and stave off hunger, but it can also contribute to water retention.

Diuretics

Taking diuretics would appear to be the obvious solution to water retention, but the relief is temporary because any kind of dehydration will cause the body to try to further retain its water reserves and make the condition worse. Furthermore, most over-the-counter diuretics deplete potassium if it is not contained in the formula, further exacerbating the condition.

Only ever take prescription diuretics under the guidance of a medical practitioner. Diuretics will lower blood pressure, and if this comes about too quickly, it is a shock to the system that may prove fatal.

Supplementation with dandelion root is useful for its diuretic and blood-purifying properties. Dandelion root is also high in potassium. Natural supplements with diuretic properties include: burdock root, corn silk, dandelion root, fennel, garlic, hibiscus, horsetail, nettle, parsley.

Drink More Water

In order to reduce water retention, dramatically increase water consumption to up to 6 liters per day, but do not drink more than a liter in an hour. The increased water consumption will cause the body to flush out its water stores, as it has no need of them.

Only consume such a large quantity of water for the purpose of curing water retention. Otherwise 2 to 3 liters per day should suffice. An excessive consumption of water at any one time can prove fatal.

Supplement with Potassium

Supplementation with potassium can help with the body's sodium/potassium balance. Potassium is contained in a large variety of foods, but you require four times as much potassium as sodium, and most diets are high in sodium and low in potassium. Potassium can also become depleted by: stress, caffeine, diarrhea (laxative abuse), vomiting (bulimia) and diuretics.

Potassium-rich foods include: cream of tartar (potassium hydrogen tartrate), almonds, pumpkin seeds, spinach, avocado, turnip, mushrooms, walnuts, coconut water, pistachios, chic peas, bananas, prunes, figs, fish, meat, poultry, eggs etc.

Supplement with Magnesium

For potassium to work, the body also needs magnesium, which is why a magnesium deficiency can also give rise to water retention. A magnesium deficiency is associated with a whole host of ailments, including: water retention, depression, migraines, chronic fatigue syndrome, asthma, hypertension, constipation, type 2 diabetes etc.

Magnesium is often depleted by the same things as potassium. If you supplement with potassium, to ensure its efficacy it is also a good idea to supplement with magnesium or consume a magnesium-rich food, such as hemp seed.

Just as sodium and potassium need to be in balance, the same is true of calcium and magnesium. Advertisers often tout a high-calcium content as something healthy, but most people are unaware that they get for too much calcium in their diet from dairy products and too little magnesium, putting the calcium/magnesium balance out of kilter. Cutting down on dairy products can therefore improve on magnesium levels, which in turn can cure a whole host of ailments.

Regular Saunas

Regular saunas will detoxify the body, reduce sodium levels and act as a diuretic. A sauna will also deplete other electrolytes, such as potassium and magnesium, but this should not be a problem if you consume nutrient-rich foods on a regular bases.

It is recommended to take no more than 2 to 3 saunas per week. Drink at least a liter of water in the sauna with added lemon or limejuice for their alkalinizing and detoxification properties. Their vitamin C content will also bolster the immune system.

Supplements for Fluid Retention:

• Water, up to 6 liters per day with added lemon or limejuice for up to 5 days.

• Vitamin B1, 500 mg per day.

• Benfotiamine (soluble B1), 300 mg up to twice per day.

• Cream of tartar (potassium hydrogen tartrate), 1 teaspoon twice per day until symptoms alleviate, then ¼ teaspoon per day thereafter.

• Potassium chloride or gluconate, 500 mg twice per day.

• Chelated magnesium, 5 mg per pound in body weight.

• Vitamin B6 (pyridoxal 5-phosphate, the biologically active form), up to 100 mg per day.

• Shelled hemp seed (high in magnesium), 1 to 2 tablespoons per day.

• Dandelion root (as a diuretic), 500 mg three times per day.

Diabetes and Fluid Retention

A common symptom of an abnormally elevated blood sugar level is fluid retention. Elevated blood sugar is highly damaging to the kidneys. Albumen is lost through the urine and blood albumen levels decline, leading to fluid retention. If you also have some of the following symptoms, you may be suffering from the early stages of diabetes:

• Foamy urine (discounting contamination with semen) caused by albumin

• Tingling in the extremities

• Poor circulation

• Occasional blurred vision

• Skin tags

• Fungal infections

• Brain fog

• Fatigue

If you believe you might be suffering the consequences of an abnormally elevated blood sugar level, moderate the medium-insulin mode, outlined in Chapter 1. Completely avoid the high-insulin mode, as well as supplements such as L-leucine and D-ribose.

It would be best to keep to a ketogenic diet and employ occasional water fasts in order to detoxify the kidneys and improve insulin sensitivity. Supplements that may help with kidney function and diabetes complications include:

• Bicarbonate of soda (US baking powder), 1 to 2 grams on an empty stomach preferably before bed.

• Acetyl L-carnitine (with biotin), 1 to 2 grams up to 3 times per day.

• Alpha lipoic acid, 600 mg up to 3 times per day.

• L-glutamine (to help elevate blood albumin), 7 grams up to 3 times per day.

• Vitamin B12, 2 to 3 mcg per day.

• Benfotiamine (fat-soluble vitamin B1), 250 mg up to 3 times per day.

• Magnesium, 1 to 3 grams per day.

• MSM (organic sulfur), 1 to 5 grams (depending on tolerance) up to twice per day.

A Sluggish Lymphatic System

Lymphedema refers to the leakage of lymph into various bodily cavities and is another form of fluid retention that is a lot more common than people realize. A clogged lymph node can cause swelling in a particular extremity, but it is more often the case that lymphedema is caused by a sluggish lymphatic system.

A sluggish lymphatic system can be brought on by a variety of things, including: acidosis, toxins, an inflammatory food allergy, sleep apnea, autoimmune poly-glandular syndrome, spontaneous bacterial peritonitis, congestive heart failure, a congenital lymphatic abnormality, impaired immune function, liver cancer and impaired liver function as a result of long-term substance abuse, alcohol abuse, steroid abuse or long-term medication etc. If you have lymphedema and wish to use a gym, it is especially important to take remedial action, as any exercise produces free radicals that can place a further burden on the lymphatic system.

Supplements for the Lymphatic System:

• Serrapeptase, 80,000 to 500,000 IU per day on an empty stomach.

• Nattokinase, 2000 to 4000 FU.

• Echinacea, 800 to 2000 mg per day for 6 to 8 weeks, then 2 weeks break.

• Lecithin (to emulsify stubborn fat in the lymphatic system) 1200 mg up to 3 times per day.

• Cranberry (to emulsify stubborn fat in the lymphatic system).

• Avoid antioxidant supplements, which can push more toxic residues into the lymphatic system.

Other useful supplements include: acidophilus, burdock root powder, calendula, fennel, turmeric, walnut leaf. Also take digestive enzymes and betaine HCL for high-protein meals.

Things that help with Lymphatic Drainage:

• Saunas to help with detoxification.

• Jacuzzi to stimulate lymphatic flow.

• Jumping on a trampoline to stimulate lymphatic flow.

• Hot and then cold showers to stimulate lymphatic flow.

• Breathing deeply.

• Epsom salt bath to help with detoxification.

• Low intensity aerobic exercise.

• Compression garments.

• Castor oil, applied topically to lower abdomen.

Food Intake:

• Anti-inflammatory foods, such as turmeric.

• Alkalinizing foods, such as figs.

• Antioxidant foods, such as red berries and beets.

• Avoid foods with known intolerances, such as lactose, gluten or coconut oil.

• Chew food properly to improve digestion.

• Eliminate processed, microwaved and GMO foods.

• Lessen overall food intake.

Chapter Seven

Key 7:
Getting the Most out of Your Workout Program

Nothing exudes youth and vitality more than physical fitness. No matter how young you may be, being physically unfit can add years to your appearance. Physical fitness is an uphill struggle as we get older and that struggle is ever steeper if bad habits are set in at an early age, but you can still get fit at any age if you have the keys.

Cardiovascular Exercise

Cardiovascular exercise will certainly burn calories, but hours of low-level cardio will also produce damaging free radicals that can wear down bodily resources that maybe detrimental to your health long term. If you are overweight with a slightly acidic body chemistry and suddenly decide to get fit, a daily routine of pounding a treadmill for an hour or so is probably the worst thing you can do to your knees and hips. A hip or knee replacement in old age is not something to look forward to.

If you think of your body as an automobile, by constantly refilling it with gasoline and pushing up the mileage, you are going to run that car into the ground. Though your body has natural recuperative qualities unlike an automobile, aerobic exercise is not intense enough to trigger a significant recuperative growth-hormone response in the same way as weight training. Hours of aerobic exercise can subject the body to a great deal of oxidative stress that may store up problems in the future, such as the onset of arthritis.

Nevertheless, if burning fat is paramount, the way to get the best out of any aerobic exercise is to perform it on an empty stomach or first thing in the morning before eating. This way, any energy expenditure during the exercises should eat straight into fat stores. Much of the research into this subject would appear to be contradictory, but ultimately it depends on your own physiology. The more often you exercise and fast, the more you train your body to utilize fat as an energy source instead of muscle tissue.

If you have been fasting, it is a good idea to coordinate any aerobic exercise toward the end of the fast. However, it is not advisable to do intense aerobic exercise on an empty stomach for more than half an hour, and it is best to eat something soon afterwards lest you should suffer the ill effects of low-blood sugar. If you wish to avoid jogging as a means of burning calories, there are plenty of alternatives that are less taxing on the knees and hips, such as walking, aerobics classes, dancing or even stomach crunches.

Stamina

Stamina nevertheless is important to health. Though there maybe pitfalls to engaging in too much aerobic exercise, that is not to suggest that those who avoid aerobic exercise altogether should feel smug, because they are likely to be lacking in stamina. If you are incapable of running flat out for at least five minutes, you have a problem.

If your body chemistry is on the acidic side, your body is unlikely to be able to make full use of oxygen, no matter how hard you train. Normalizing your acid/alkaline body chemistry by changing your diet should go a long way to improving the utilization of oxygen and improving stamina.

Supplementation with the amino acid, HMB, will not only reduce metabolic acidosis, but will improve aerobic performance by increasing VO2 max (maximal oxygen consumption). Regular, intensive cardiovascular exercise will also raise your blood-oxygen levels by training your body to use oxygen more efficiently. It will improve circulation, lung capacity and heart function.

To improve stamina, set goals for yourself and regularly improve upon these goals until you have achieved the level of stamina you desire. From then on, you will need only to perform this level of intensive aerobic exercise in brief bursts a few times a week to maintain your capacity. Regular short bursts of intensive aerobic exercise is just as effective at maintaining a high level of stamina as daily routines of hours of low-intensity aerobic work, as long as you do not shock the body with anything too strenuous.

Keep in mind that to be in great shape, you need only the potential to be able to perform. You do not need to run several miles a day to prove the point, and if you did so, you would probably do more harm than good.

To sum up, do not bother with laborious jogging or pounding on the treadmill. Replace this with a few short bursts of intensive aerobic activity per week to maintain stamina. Try several 30-second bursts of high-intensity aerobic activity, allowing yourself a few minutes rest in between to get your breath back.

Alternatively, a one-minute all-out sprint on a treadmill each time you visit the gym may well suffice. This might not seem much, but a one-minute sprint on a track can take you quite a distance. This can be combined with long walks or any other form of low-intensity aerobic exercise that is not too taxing on the joints.

IGF-1

IGF-1 (Insulin-Like Growth Factor 1) is an endogenous molecule synthesized primarily in the liver using insulin and growth hormone. A study published in *The Journal of Clinical Endocrinology*, Oct 1996, shows that short-duration, high-intensity exercise, such as weight training or a short, all-out sprint, increases IGF-1 levels far more effectively than other forms of exercise.

IGF-1 has been noted for its effect on muscle mass and strength, as well as its ability to repair damaged cells. For these reasons, IGF-1 is considered an anti-aging molecule, and because of its ability to mimic the effects of insulin, increased IGF-1 levels can also help with the symptoms of diabetes.

Supplements that increase IGF-1 levels include whey protein and the amino acid, creatine. Whey protein can be consumed in a shake once or twice a day, and creatine can be taken as a supplement in a recommended dose of 5 grams a day with no adverse side effects apart from a slight elevation in DHT levels.

Weight Training

Weight training or anaerobic exercise is primarily used to increase muscle mass, though it is also an effective means of losing body fat. Greater muscle mass will not only make you look fitter and younger, but will also speed up your metabolism, making dieting easier. Though weight training produces free radicals, it is far better at triggering bodily repair mechanisms than aerobic exercise.

Apart from diet, the key to anaerobic exercise is rest. If you weight train every muscle group every day, you may burn calories, but you will over train and not grow. It is only during the rest period that muscles have the chance to recuperate and grow, and each muscle group requires at least a week to recover. The older you are, the more recovery time you will need, and you may require up to three weeks rest for each muscle group. Every 6 to 8 weeks it is advisable to take a complete week rest from training in order to ensure that the body recovers properly.

Another important factor is training intensity. Push every muscle group to muscle failure at the end of each set and rest for three minutes between each set. The aim of weight training is to induce small tears along the length of a muscle to cause it to grow.

However, it is important not to get into a routine. Always try new exercises and routines in order to shock the muscles, but never exercise through pain. If you have any injury, no matter how minor, you must rest, otherwise you will set yourself up for a far worse injury and an even longer recuperation time that may require medical intervention.

If you have incorporated fasting into your routine, your body will increase the production of HGH and recovery times should reduce. During a fast, growth hormone naturally peaks toward the end of the fast. Given that weight training also stimulates the production of growth hormone, it is a good idea to coordinate a workout at the end of a fast for maximum growth-hormone production.

Gym Routine

If a cold muscle is suddenly made to perform a heavy lifting action, it may tear, requiring a great amount of recovery time, setting you back considerably with your training. For this reason always start with a warm-up set with a low weight for each exercise.

However, it is not good practice to begin your training routine with stretch exercises. If your muscles are over stretched, this will hamper your performance when it comes to lifting heavy weights. Reserve the stretch exercises for the end of the routine for the purpose of maintaining suppleness. A few yoga positions should suffice.

A 5 or 6-way split routine, focusing on each individual muscle group each day, is designed for professional bodybuilders who use anabolic steroids. Massive gains are achieved because anabolic steroids reduce recover times.

A 3-way split training routine with four days rest should suffice for most people unless you are genetically predisposed to being fit. Given that the chest muscles work with the triceps, and the back muscles work with the biceps, a 3-way split will prevent you from working the same muscle groups two days running.

However, if time is precious, it is feasible to exercise the whole body in one day and rest for six days if every muscle group is pushed to the limit. If you are starting out as a weight trainer, instead of laboriously heading to the gym everyday in a desperate effort to get in shape, this is probably all you need to do for the first few months to adapt your body to a weight-training regimen. Remember that rest is even more important than the actual muscle exertion for the purpose of gaining muscle.

Three-Day Routine

• Day 1: biceps and back

• Day 2: chest, shoulders and triceps

• Day 3: legs

Sets and Reps

The purpose of a warm-up set is to prepare your muscles for the heavier sets. Each exercise should consist of 3 to 5 sets:

• A warm-up set of 20 to 30 reps

• A heavier set of 15 to 20 reps

• Two heavy sets of 10 to 12 reps

• A final heavy set of 8 to 10 reps

The Burn

To increase the intensity of a workout routine, upon each oscillation, stop half way before continuing. Make your muscles do the work instead of relying upon the momentum of the weight. On the final few reps, you may work a complete oscillation.

In the final set, you should achieve muscle-overload. To get the maximum from your last set, try pumping the weight on the last rep with several small oscillations to give your muscles what is termed a burn. Once muscle-overload is achieved on your final heavy set, continuing to work this muscle or muscle group serves no purpose and may lead to injury.

Things to Avoid at the Health Club:

• Exercise vibration plates advertise themselves as a shortcut to toning up muscles. However, there have been no studies as to their long-term impact on health. These machines will certainly vibrate muscle tissue, but they will also vibrate your spinal chord and your brain. Any vibration of the brain is likely to cause it to swell, killing brain cells in the process. This is likely to lead to memory loss and symptoms of Alzheimer's dementia.

• The Jacuzzi is an ideal way to relax after an exercise routine and to stimulate lymphatic flow, but a high-power jet of water directed against your upper body will also vibrate the brain with similar consequences as the exercise vibration plate. If you use a Jacuzzi, it is better to avoid a jet hitting the upper spine for any length of time.

• Saunas offer the user an extremely sterile environment because of the intense heat, but the same cannot be said of a steam room with its warm, moisture-laden air. It is possible to pick up a bacterial infection such as pneumonia from a steam room if it is not well maintained. Even if a steam room is well looked after, if you share this space with anybody with an illness, the steam-room environment can be a hot house for passing on a contagion.

• Sun beds are often used to compensate for a working life of air-conditioned offices throughout most of the daylight hours of the year, but there are few things more damaging to the skin than a sun bed. Though sun beds will stimulate what appears to be a healthy glow, they have been referred to as time machines for their ability to age the skin prematurely.

A sun bed may be useful for the purpose of building up some sun protection to prevent burning under natural sunlight if a holiday is planned. Otherwise, for those who are pale-skinned and looking for a tan, begin sunbathing daily under natural sunlight for ten to fifteen minutes for the first few days and build up the amount of time spent in the sun over successive weeks.

Using sunscreen will simply lengthen exposure to the most harmful rays. It is far better to forego sunscreen and to be out in the sun for far shorter periods of time. Sunscreen is ideally used as protection if you must be out in the sun for long stretches or if you wish to protect the face, neck and hands on a daily basis from the aging effects of strong sunlight, though supplementation with vitamin D3 is advised.

Chapter Eight

A Glossary of Useful Super Foods

The obesity problem of today and most of today's ailments are a product of a modern diet high in sugar and processed foods, not to mention the relatively recent introduction of genetically modified foods. Widespread ailments associated with a modern Western diet include: obesity, heart disease, high blood pressure, diabetes, asthma, allergies, IBS, arthritis, sleep apnea, Alzheimer's disease etc.

However, instead of pointing the finger at new innovations in food production, scientists, until quite recently, singled out as problematic foods that we have been consuming for thousands of years, such as: eggs, butter, cheese and meat. Moreover it is not the cholesterol that is the problem with any of these foods but the way in which most of the farm animals today are reared to produce them.

Nevertheless, just because a food is deemed healthy does not mean it will be good for you if you are not used to digesting it. Too much of such a food may well go undigested and ferment in the gut and give rise to even more toxins than the junk food you are used to.

After a bad reaction to a certain food in the digestive tract, subsequently even small amounts could give rise to an autoimmune response. The body has a memory and thinks it is under attack. Therefore, it is always advisable to introduce new foods into your diet gradually and to increase the portions in stages over several weeks.

There are an enumerable number of foods that can be called super foods. This is a compilation of foods that are not by any means the only super foods, but this list should give you an idea of the power of food.

Açaí berries are an important part of the diet of peoples throughout the Amazon region. They are noted mostly for their antioxidant properties, which have powerful anti-aging properties. They are high in vitamins, minerals, fiber and many other compounds beneficial to health.

At present, fresh açaí berries are only available in parts of South America such as Brazil. Açaí products are available in other parts of the world derived from frozen açaí pulp.

Always choose a product that has undergone the least amount of processing in order that its health properties are maximized. Spray-dried açaí or açaí extract are best avoided. Some of the health properties attributed to the açaí berry include:

• Açaí increases energy levels and stamina.
• It has the ability to lower bad cholesterol whilst increasing good cholesterol levels.
• It is high in vitamin C, improving immunity.
• It has anti-inflammatory properties, helping with such ailments as arthritis.
• It promotes a healthy heart.
• Consumption of açaí is noted for making skin radiant and the hair lustrous.

Almonds are considered the most nutritious of nuts and are one of the few nuts that are alkaline forming. They are high in protein and fiber but low in carbohydrate.

Almonds are loaded with vitamin E and other antioxidants. They contain many B vitamins and are high in minerals such as magnesium, potassium, calcium and iron.

Almonds are best consumed raw as roasted almonds can lose many of their nutritive properties. The health benefits of almonds include:
• 66% of the fat in almonds is monounsaturated, making almonds a useful food for lowering LDL cholesterol.
• A study has shown a link between the consumption of nuts, and especially almonds, and a reduced risk of contracting chronic diseases such as cancer, Alzheimer's disease and diabetes.
• Though almonds are high in calories, they also contain phenylalanine, which is an appetite suppressant. A few almonds can stave off the hunger or make you less inclined to overeat at mealtimes.

Apple Cider vinegar has long been used in folk remedy for all manner of ailments. It has the unique property of being the only vinegar that is alkaline forming when digested. It is useful to dieters because it lowers an insulin spike.

Cider vinegar can be used as a condiment or used with olive oil as a salad dressing. You can also add two tablespoons of cider vinegar to an herbal tea half an hour before a meal, but do not be tempted to drink it neat, as the acid can corrode the enamel of your teeth as well as sensitize your gums and the lining of your throat. Excessive intake of apple cider vinegar can deplete potassium.

Always buy the raw, unfiltered, organic cider vinegar rather than cheaper pasteurized versions. Its many health properties include:
• Cider vinegar is useful to dieters for its ability to reduce appetite and speed up the metabolism. It lowers glucose levels and reduces an insulin spike after a carbohydrate-rich meal. An insulin spike not only puts the body in fat-storing mode, but will make you feel tired. Consume 2 tablespoons in water half an hour before every meal.
• It can help those suffering from type 2 diabetes because of its ability to help level out blood sugar levels.
• It helps with digestion by working as a corrective agent for the amount of acid your stomach produces. It may reduce the symptoms of acid reflux, mild heartburn and gastro-esophageal reflux disease.
• Its amino acid content makes it an agent for controlling cholesterol.
• Diluted with water, cider vinegar can be applied topically and used as a toner to help with skin complaints such as acne.

Artichoke is one of the few vegetables that can be bought in supplement form, such are its nutritive properties. Artichoke is high in vitamins, minerals and fiber as well many other natural health-promoting compounds.

If you are at a loss as to what to do with artichoke, which is not a simple vegetable to prepare, artichoke hearts can be purchased as an antipasto and simply added to a salad. Other health properties of artichoke include:
• Artichoke is prized for its effect on liver function, protecting against toxins and infection. Artichoke, especially the leaves, increases bile secretion, helping with digestion, which is most useful for people suffering from irritable bowel syndrome.
• It reduces LDL cholesterol levels.
• Fresh artichoke can help stabilize blood-sugar levels in diabetes.

Black Cumin can be purchased as seeds or as an oil. Apart from its use as a culinary spice, it has long been used for medicinal purposes since ancient times and is often referred to as a panacea:
• Black cumin helps fight disease by boosting the immune system.
• It has been shown to be effective in combating autoimmune disorders.
• It has anti-cancer properties and may be used in conjunction with conventional therapies in the treatment of cancer.
• It is an anti-inflammatory and may help in the treatment of respiratory diseases, rheumatism and arthritis.
• It can act as an adaptogen by increasing energy levels, help alleviate depression and calm the nervous system.
• It can help alleviate or prevent high blood pressure.
• It may be used as a digestive aid and quell colic pain, constipation, flatulence, diarrhea, dysentery and hemorrhoids.

• Black cumin may be used by women to stimulate menstrual periods or increase the flow of milk for nursing mothers.

Blue cheese, like any cheese, becomes a super food when it is aged and made from unpasteurized milk. Good quality cheeses are one of the best sources of probiotics, an important constituent to a healthy diet. Blue cheese also has anti-inflammatory properties.

Regular consumption of blue cheese is believed to be one of the reasons why the French enjoy better health than other Europeans. France's most famous blue cheese, Roquefort, which is made from ewe's milk, is called the cheese of kings and popes.

Ewe's or goat's cheese may be preferred by those with an intolerance to cow's milk. Otherwise, the many health properties of blue cheese include:
• The probiotics of blue cheese help with gastrointestinal health, Candida, yeast infections, allergies and food intolerances.
• An improved immune system can stave off cold and flu.
• Its anti-inflammatory properties can help with cardiovascular disease and arthritis.
• Cheese has a high CLA content that can help with weight loss if part of a balanced diet.

Burdock root can be consumed as a vegetable, a spice or taken in supplement form. Burdock root is an ancient remedy to purify the blood and cool internal heat. It detoxifies the blood, the lymphatic system and the skin. It has powerful anti-inflammatory properties, as well as anti-oxidant, anti-bacterial and anti-cancer properties.

Burdock root can re-grow damaged liver cells and can help expel gallstones. It stimulates blood circulation to the skin. It has expectorant and decongestant properties. It is a diuretic and helps induce lymphatic drainage and detoxification. It contains inulin, a soluble prebiotic fibre, that can help lower blood sugar levels.

Fresh burdock root, which is used in many Asian dishes, is probably not easy to find. In powdered form, which can be ordered on line, it can be added to soups or made into a tea. In supplement form, take 3 g up to three times per day. Consuming burdock root can help with the following:
• Burdock root can be taken to treat or prevent a variety of cancers.
• Its anti-inflammatory properties can help with many conditions including arthritis and fibromyalgia.
• Its anti-bacterial properties can help with most skin conditions.
• Its detoxification properties can help with liver cirrhosis, bile production, digestion and weight loss.
• Its diuretic properties can help with fluid retention, as well as reducing sodium.
• It can help with diabetes and diabetes complications.

Cayenne pepper, as a culinary spice, is a constituent of many recipes. It is a favorite with dieters for its ability to speed up the metabolism. The many health benefits of cayenne pepper include:
• It not only stimulates an artificial fever that boosts the fight against the flu virus, but also helps alleviate mucus congestion.
• It is a digestive aid that speeds digestion and increases the flow of digestive enzymes and gastric juices, and is useful as part of a weight-loss program.
• It is a strong anti-inflammatory that can help with arthritis.
• It neutralizes acidity.
• It stimulates circulation and speeds up the metabolism to help with weight loss.
• It has detoxifying and anti-fungal properties that can help with gastrointestinal health.
• It normalizes blood pressure and reduces bad cholesterol.

Cinnamon is another culinary spice with many health benefits favored by dieters for its ability to lower an insulin spike. Ceylon cinnamon is preferable to regular cassia cinnamon, which can be toxic when used in large quantities over a long period of time.

Half a teaspoon a day is recommended and can be added to a cup of herbal tea. The many health benefits of cinnamon include:
• In a study in 'The American Journal of Clinical Nutrition' (2007) seasoning a high carbohydrate meal with cinnamon helped avoid an insulin spike. Cinnamon also appears to normalize blood sugar levels in people suffering from type 2 diabetes by improving insulin sensitivity.
• It is a powerful anti-bacterial agent that can be used to stop the growth of Candida or yeast infections in the gut.
• Cinnamon is known for its ability to boost brain function for anybody concerned about cognitive decline and is also known for its anti-inflammatory properties.
• Studies have shown cinnamon supplementation to increase testosterone levels in men.

Coconut oil is rich in medium-chain triglycerides or MCTs, which are easily digested to provides ketones as a source of energy, notably to the brain, without being stored as body fat. Coconut oil makes an excellent cooking oil whereby its health properties take away the guilt of eating fried food.

It is always advisable to introduce coconut oil slowly to the diet, as it may not be tolerated by some people, as it can be highly inflammatory. Never buy hydrogenated coconut oil.

Caprylic acid, which is an MCT derived from coconut oil, may be preferable to coconut oil for the treatment of Candida or Alzheimer's dementia. Adding coconut oil to your diet can help with the following:
• Coconut oil's anti-fungal properties can help with Candida overgrowth.
• It is noted for its anti-fungal, antiviral and antibacterial properties.

• It's high MCT oil content can help with endurance, mental performance and Alzheimer's dementia.
• It's MCT oil content can help with insulin resistance because it escorts sugar into the cells without insulin.
• It is an appetite suppressant, will speed the metabolism and help with weight loss.
• It can help with Parkinson's disease.
• Its anti-viral properties can help with all manner of viral infection.
• Coconut oil's cholesterol profile is good for boosting testosterone and balancing hormones.

Cranberries are known for their curative power with regard to urinary tract infections because of their antibacterial properties. Cranberries are most likely purchased as a juice, but choose a product without preservatives or added sugar if possible.

For the maximum benefit from cranberries, it is always best to consume a product that has undergone the least amount of processing. The health benefits of cranberries include:
• Regular consumption of cranberries can offer a natural alternative to some prescription antibiotics and can even be used against strains of antibiotic-resistant bacteria.
• Cranberry is a digestive aid and emulsifies stubborn fat in the lymphatic system, helping with the immune system, amongst other things.
• It can help prevent a stroke or heart attack by making hardened arteries more flexible by removing plaque build-up in arterial walls.
• It has anti-inflammatory properties and may help with the treatment of inflammatory diseases such as rheumatoid arthritis.
• Laboratory studies have shown extracts of cranberry to inhibit the growth of cancerous tumors.

Eggs are not often regarded as a super food because of their high cholesterol content, but most foods that are close to the origins of life, such as nuts and fruits, offer a highly concentrated form of nutrition. For those concerned about the high cholesterol content of eggs, the high lecithin content more than negates any negative effect.

Eggs are packed with fats, proteins, minerals and vitamins, especially B vitamins, notably choline, which is important to brain function. The only downside of consuming a large amount of eggs is that they may be constipating, especially if hardboiled. Always consume eggs with some form of roughage.

Eggs are inexpensive and readily available, but the more expensive varieties tend to have the highest nutritional value. Eating eggs can be helpful for the following:
• The high vitamin B content can lower anxiety and depression.

• The high choline content can help with brain function, memory and Alzheimer's disease.
• Eggs are an excellent source of high quality protein and can help with weight loss.
• The high lecithin content of eggs can on balance lower cholesterol.

Figs are an ideal food to counter many of the ill effects of our modern diet: insulin insensitivity, high cholesterol, hypertension, potassium depletion, an acidic body PH and constipation. Packed with antioxidants, vitamins, minerals and fiber, the health benefits of figs are many:
• Figs are sweet but do not produce an insulin spike. Their high potassium content lowers blood sugar levels and will lower the insulin requirement for people suffering from diabetes.
• The high potassium content of figs should redress potassium depletion caused by excessive consumption of coffee, as well as a diet high in sodium.
• Fresh Figs in particular help regulate the body's PH because they are one of the most alkaline-forming foods.
• Figs are a mild laxative and contain both fiber and soluble fiber, making them the ideal food to deal with constipation, another common problem with the modern diet. The soluble fiber in figs can also help lower LDL cholesterol and help eliminate the body of toxins.

Garlic has long been used medicinally in Europe for a variety of ailments. It will not only help lower cholesterol levels, it helps dilate blood vessels as well as being a potent blood thinner. Its anti-inflammatory and antioxidant properties protect blood vessels from the build up of plaque and unwanted clogging. All these properties make garlic an indispensible food to help lower high blood pressure, help with heart disease and prevent a stroke.

Notwithstanding its effect on the breath, a too large quantity of raw garlic in your diet can be toxic. Garlic can be consumed in much larger quantities when cooked, dried, powdered, pickled or aged. Never store garlic in oil at room temperature, as the sulphurous nature of garlic makes this a breeding ground for botulism. Garlic's many health properties include:
• Garlic has anti-inflammatory properties, helping with diseases like asthma and rheumatoid arthritis.
• It helps control blood sugar and is therefore useful to people that are insulin resistant.
• It has strong antibacterial, antimicrobial and antiviral properties. It can even help treat bacterial infections that have become resistant to prescription antibiotics.
• It gives the immune system a boost by stimulating white blood cells. Together with its antioxidant properties, this has the added bonus of reducing the risk of many forms of cancer. Research has suggested that a diet with a high intake of garlic reduces all forms of cancer (apart from prostate and breast cancer).

• Packed with antioxidants, such as selenium, garlic is known for its anti-aging properties.

Gelatin is an inexpensive and much-ignored super food with a variety of health benefits. Gelatin simply the cooked form of collagen, which is the most abundant protein in the human body.

Gelatin can be bought as a powder and added to soups, deserts or any hot beverage. It is used in many commercial products as a thickener. Bone broth is a rich source of gelatin that also has a high mineral content.

As a food supplement, begin with 2 tablespoons of gelatin powder per day and build up to 6 tablespoons. Consumption of gelatin can help with the following:
• Its collagen-boosting properties are anti-aging and can help with skin, hair and nails.
• Collagen plays an important role in many bodily functions: it is essential to skin elasticity and the appearance of youth and is an essential nutrient to all connective tissues.
• Gelatin is an anti-inflammatory and is useful in healing, growth, the prevention of allergies and digestive health.
• It may help normalize gut hormones in people with obesity.
• It can help with brain function and Alzheimer's disease.
• It has anti-estrogenic properties.
• It can help with autoimmune diseases: allergies, arthritis, asthma etc.
• Its water solubility can help with constipation.
• It can normalize blood sugar and help with diabetes.
• It can stimulate growth hormone production.
• It can heal the gut and help with: leaky gut, IBS, immune health, inflammatory bowel disease etc.
• It can help with insomnia.
• It can help with joint and bone health, as well as arthritis.
• It can help with weight loss.
• It can help with wound healing.

Hemp seeds are considered the most nutritious of any seed. They are a concentrated source of protein, essential fatty acids, vitamins, minerals, enzymes and fiber, but contain virtually no carbohydrates or saturated fats. They are classified as a complete protein.

If you are seeking a cheap alternative to a variety of costly supplements, shelled hemp seeds may provide the answer. Many of the health benefits of hemp seeds are attributed to its high magnesium content.

Shelled hemp seeds can be added to smoothies, breakfast cereals or simply eaten on its own. The enumerable health benefits of shelled hemp seeds include:
• Hemp seed has anti-inflammatory properties.
• It can help reduce cholesterol and blood pressure.

• It improves circulation.
• I bolsters the immune system.
• It can strengthen hair, skin and nails.
• It can help with intestinal problems and constipation
• It can help with weight loss and water retention etc.

Honey/manuka honey (raw/unpasteurized) have been used for its healing properties for centuries. It is high in antioxidants and digestive enzymes. Like vitamin C, honey is a precursor to hydrogen peroxide, which increases blood oxygen.

A good honey should have a strength level of around 3. Manuka honey can be anything between strength level 5 and 20. Always buy a honey with its strength level labeled, as processed honey can contain no useful therapeutic properties whatsoever. The health benefits of raw honey are many:
• An elevated blood oxygen level will bolster the immune system by killing viruses, bacteria, fungi and even cancer cells.
• It contains bee pollen which can provide natural allergy relief and bolster the immune system.
• Used as a sweetener, compared to refined sugar, honey is alkaline forming and has a lower glycemic index, which can help with weight loss.
• It can increase alertness and give you greater stamina. For this reason, manuka honey is often used by athletes.
• It provides an easily absorbed supply of carbohydrate in the form of liver glycogen, making it a healthier option for athletes than energy drinks.
• Honey can also be applied topically to treat wounds and bacterial infection. As soon as honey comes into contact with skin, a chemical reaction occurs that brings about the slow release of hydrogen peroxide.

Fermented foods were part of most staple diets until relatively recently. Traditionally, foods were fermented to naturally extend their shelf life. A fermented food is rich in vitamin K2, friendly flora and digestive enzymes that are vital to the digestive tract and to good health.

Fermented foods include: live yoghurt, crème fraiche, aged cheese, sauerkraut, fermented tofu, sprouted foods, bresaola, prosciutto and traditionally fermented soy products such as soy sauce and misu etc. However the pasteurization of many commercial products completely negates many of the health benefits that a fermented food might offer. The benefits of fermented foods include:
• Fermented foods increase the digestibility of other foods.
• They increase in alkalinity and neutralize body pH levels.
• They boost to the immune system.
• They increase friendly bacterial in the gut and help with gastrointestinal health.
• Fermented foods help eliminate toxins from the body etc.

• The high vitamin K2 content helps with vitamin D3 absorption.

Ginger has long been used medicinally in the East for gastrointestinal relief and to alleviate symptoms of irritable bowl syndrome. Ginger can be added as a spice to a large number of recipes from cakes to curries or used to make a tea.

Fresh ginger is highly concentrated in active substances and very little of it is needed for medicinal use. The health benefits of ginger include:
• Ginger is effective in reducing the symptoms of motion sickness: nausea, dizziness and cold sweats. It can also help with morning sickness in pregnant women without the side effects of anti-vomiting drugs, which can cause birth defects.
• It helps eliminate gas and has a calming effect on the intestinal tract.
• It has potent anti-inflammatory properties that can help with the pain of rheumatoid arthritis.
• It has antioxidant and anti-cancer properties.
• It has immune boosting properties.

Licorice root is an herb mostly known as a candy flavoring, though some commercial licorice is actually flavored with anise. Licorice root is an adaptogen, a stimulant and a powerful anti-inflammatory.

Licorice root has phytoestrogen properties beneficial to women's health and anti-DHT properties that help prevent male-pattern baldness. It is most notable for treating adrenal fatigue and gastrointestinal problems such as leaky gut.

Licorice root can be bought as a powder and added to smoothies or teas as a flavoring. Do not consume more than one level teaspoon twice a day, otherwise over stimulation can cause a headache.

Prolonged use of licorice root can raise blood pressure and it is not advisable to use it every day for more than two weeks at a time. Because of its estrogen-like effect on women, pregnant women should not consume licorice root. Consumption of licorice root can help with the following:
• It regulates cortisol, the stress hormone, helping with adrenal fatigue and endurance.
• Its anti-inflammatory properties can help with leaky gut syndrome and help heal ulcers.
• It is an effective treatment for acid reflux, indigestion and stomach pain.
• It has antiviral properties that can be used to counter all manner of infections, including HIV, Hepatitis C and influenza.
• It is an effective expectorant and useful for treating rhinitis and colds.
• It has an estrogen-like effect on women and can be used for PMS and menopause symptoms.
• It acts as a hydrocortisone and can be used for pain relief.
• Its anti-DHT properties can promote hair growth.

• Applied topically, it can be used to help remove hyper-pigmentation, stimulate hair growth and help with pain relief.

Olive oil is a staple of the Mediterranean diet and its health properties are numerous. All types of olive oil are good sources of monounsaturated fat, but extra virgin olive oil, which is the first cold press of the olives, contains the greatest number of health properties when consumed raw.

Glass containers are preferable to plastic containers given that plastic is likely to adulterate the olive oil over time with estrogen-mimicking petro-chemicals. Always store olive oil in a cool place away from sunlight, as heat and sunlight can cause it to go rancid.

Do not waste your olive oil on frying. When it is exposed to high heat, it changes into harmful trans fats. For frying, use rapeseed oil or a saturated fat like butter or coconut oil. The benefits of raw, extra virgin olive oil include:

• Extra virgin olive oil will reduce LDL cholesterol and reduce the risk of coronary heart disease.

• It has been found to contain a naturally occurring chemical that protects brain cells from neurotoxins responsible for Alzheimer's disease and brain damage.

• It expels poisons and intestinal parasites from the digestive tract.

• It feeds good bacteria to help with digestion and undermines the ability of bad bacteria such as Candida to take a hold.

• It will speed up the digestive system and ease constipation, as well as offer benefits in colon cancer prevention.

• It will ward off diseases of the respiratory tract such as pleurisy, bronchitis, pneumonia and the common cold.

• It stimulates the production of bile and pancreatic hormones to help with gastrointestinal functions and will consequently reduce the production of gallbladder stones.

• It can also be used to expel gallbladder stones.

• Olive oil in your diet will give a healthy glow to your complexion and make your hair more lustrous.

• It can be used to help with the skin complaints, psoriasis and eczema, and is highly effective against dandruff. The application of olive oil to the scalp is an ancient remedy for alopecia.

• Applied topically, olive oil can be used to ward off skin infections such as ringworm.

Organ meats may not be considered a super food, but for meat eaters, organ meats are by far the most nutritious part of the animal. Organ meats are packed with vitamins, minerals, amino acids and many compounds beneficial to health. Common organ meats include: liver, kidney, heart, brain and sweetbreads.

Consumption of a particular organ meat can be used to treat a corresponding organ malady. Supplements made from dried animal organ meat, called glandulars, are widely used for their remarkable therapeutic benefits.

Grass-fed meat is preferable to standard, commercially produced meat. If you like eating meat, organ meats make a cheaper and far more nutritious alternative to regular meat.

Parsley has been used medicinally since ancient times. It is part of the same family of herbs as gotu kola, and like gotu kola can be used to enhance brain function and improve memory.

Parsley has a high vitamin and mineral content. Large amounts of parsley can also be added to a salad if chopped up finely. The health benefits of parsley include:

• Parsley strengthens the immune system and works as a decongestant; it is therefore useful to take if you are suffering from cold or flu.

• It can help treat digestive disorders and reduce bloating.

• It can help regulate blood sugar.

• It has anti-inflammatory properties and can help alleviate the pain of various types of arthritis.

• It is one of the most effective natural diuretics.

• It can lower blood pressure, help with cardiovascular diseases and prevent stroke.

• It contains antioxidants that neutralize certain carcinogens, therefore helping to prevent the onset or spread of cancer.

Turmeric is a versatile spice with many properties for good health. Principal of these is its ability to improve memory and help prevent Alzheimer's dementia. In India, where turmeric is much used in food, the incidence of Alzheimer's disease is a quarter of that of the US.

The main active component of turmeric is curcumin. The absorption of curcumin is helped by the presence of piperine, a component of black pepper, which is often combined with turmeric in Indian cuisine.

A build up of plaque in the brain triggers inflammation that kills brain cells and gives rise to Alzheimer's dementia. Turmeric works in a twofold manner by helping clear away this plaque and act as an anti-inflammatory.

Turmeric lowers fibrinogen levels to help with cardiovascular disease, diabetes and even scarring. It also contains many anti-oxidants and has anti-carcinogenic properties.

If you are not a fan of Indian food, turmeric's nutty flavor and color lends itself to any rice dish, mashed potatoes and even to popcorn. You can consume up to 3.8 grams per day without any adverse effects. Its many health-giving properties include:

• Turmeric's anti-inflammatory properties can also help with arthritis, Alzheimer's disease and congestive heart failure.

• It increases liver function.

• It helps lower cholesterol.

Whey protein has an 80% protein content, which is one of the highest protein contents of any food, but many may not realize that whey protein is a super food with many remarkable health-giving properties. The top food for maximizing glutathione, which is the body's master antioxidant, is high-quality whey protein.

Whey protein is one of the very few sources of protein that is mildly alkaline forming. It also contains many amino acids useful to muscle protein synthesis.

Whey protein naturally increases IGF-1 levels (insulin-like growth factor 1) which helps with muscle mass and strength. It also slows the production of the stress hormone, cortisol, which is a catabolic hormone.

Most commercial shakes containing whey protein also contain artificial sweeteners, flavors and coloring. If you would prefer to avoid these artificial additives, buy pure whey protein powder and make your own shake. Apart from shakes and smoothies, whey protein can also be added to many baked recipes, such as waffles or quick breads.

Though whey protein is already low in lactose, if you suffer from lactose intolerance, whey protein isolate is virtually lactose free and has a 90% protein content, but as a processed product, it is not likely to have as many health benefits. Whey protein's many remarkable health-giving properties include:

• Whey protein is a favorite with bodybuilders and dieters for its ability to build or maintain muscle mass and reduce body fat.

• It is an excellent source of essential amino acids, which play an important part in the growth and repair of every aspect of human tissue, as well as body fluids, teeth, nails and hair. The promotion of skin growth can help with wound healing.

• IGF-1 mimics the effect of insulin and can help with diabetes.

• It has the ability to reduce the glucose absorption time into the bloodstream, preventing hunger and helping with type-2 diabetes.

• It helps release serotonin, which promotes a feeling of wellbeing.

• Its ability to raise glutathione will improve longevity, detoxify the body and improve immune function.

Chapter Nine

A Glossary of Useful Supplements

Many hold to the belief that supplements are not needed by anybody on a healthy diet, and this is certainly true for most people under the age of 30, but anybody older than that has been exposed to many years of environmental toxins, processed foods and various innovations of the pharmaceutical industry, not to mention over-the-counter painkillers, anabolic steroids and recreational drugs.

With the huge array of supplements available, it is always best to be highly knowledgeable about what you are taking lest you do more damage than good. It is not uncommon for a health enthusiast to take far too many supplements.

Not all dietary supplements are as well regulated as medicines, and manufacturers of supplements are motivated by profit just like Big Pharma. Unless a supplement is produced by a reliable company, it is always preferable to buy supplements in liquid, powdered or capsule form rather than tablet form. It is not uncommon for tablets to pass through the alimentary canal without being digested. Most supplements also contain binders such as magnesium stearate, which may have adverse side effects in high doses.

When choosing an herbal supplement, take note as to whether the capsules contain an herbal extract or powdered form. The milligram weight should be shown in terms of the herb's active extract. Tablets or capsules containing a highly processed powdered herb may be of little medicinal value. Otherwise buy the herb loose in its unadulterated form from a reputable source.

Amino acids can be purchased in powdered form in bulk at very reasonably prices mainly because they are popular with bodybuilders. Many overlook these supplements because of the assumption that they are only of benefit to bodybuilding, but most amino acids have remarkable medicinal properties.

Commercial bodybuilding products containing artificial flavorings and sweeteners are best avoided however.

Antioxidant Supplements

A good diet containing high levels of natural antioxidants can be shown to have many health benefits, but if you supplement with antioxidants long term to compensate for a bad diet, you may be doing more damage than good. If you have a sluggish lymphatic system or suffer from lymphedema, antioxidants are known to push more toxic residues into the lymphatic system, which operates as the body's sewer system, and worsen the condition.

Antioxidants have been noted for their anti-aging properties and were assumed to reduce the incidence of cancer, given that they mop up damaging, carcinogenic free radicals, but as the word suggests, an antioxidant inhibits oxidation, which can impair the immune system, as the body utilizes the oxidative power of hydrogen peroxide (oxygen water or H2O2) not only to fight infection, but also to kill cancer cells.

Unlike antioxidant supplements, natural foods with antioxidant properties are usually alkaline forming, and an alkaline body chemistry has a positive effect on the retention of oxygen in tissue. Therefore the net effect of these foods is to increase the body's oxygen reserves.

Trials with antioxidants have shown supplementation in many instances to increase rather than decrease the incidence of cancer. A French study involving adult females in the *Journal of National Cancer Institute* (Sept 2005) found that the non-smokers of the control group with high levels of beta-carotene had a lower risk of developing cancer than those with low levels of beta-carotene, but conversely, smokers with high levels of beta-carotene had a significantly higher risk of developing smoking-related cancers than the other smokers in the control group. Further research revealed that the high level of beta-carotene amongst the smokers in the control group was nearly always due to supplementation rather than food intake.

The antioxidant vitamin C, however, is a precursor to hydrogen peroxide. If you are supplementing with any antioxidant for any particular health condition, it is advisable to also supplement with vitamin C in a dose raging between 1000 to 2000 mg up to three times per day.

Generally, you should only supplement with antioxidants for short periods as part of a program of detoxification or if you have an ailment that might be helped by a specific supplement that contains antioxidant properties. If you succumb to any type of illness, such as a cold, it is advisable to desist from taking most antioxidant supplements apart from vitamin C in order to bolster the immune system. Supplements that help increase blood oxygen include: aloe vera, vitamin C, calcium, cordyceps, vitamin E, ginseng, iron, magnesium.

What are the Best Supplements to Take?

There are an enumerable number of supplements available and only a fraction of them are listed below. The purpose of the following list is to highlight those supplements that are likely to improve athletic performance, contribute to weight loss or are most likely to be deficient in the general population.

Never take a supplement without first doing your homework. Minerals, especially, need to be in balance with each other. Taking a specific mineral supplement can put other minerals out of kilter, which is why it is often better to supplement with food supplements, which contain a good balance of various nutrients.

It is easy to spend a large sum of money on supplements that do not appear to make much difference. For anybody over the age of 35, the following supplements should be transformative: pregnenolone, L-taurine, MSM and evening primrose oil.

Always take the recommended dose. Taking a high dose will not reverse a condition any quicker but may cause further complications.

If you are taking any type of prescription medication or have a severe medical condition, it is advisable to consult your medical practitioner before taking any dietary supplement.

Pregnant or lactating women should always consult with their doctor before taking any dietary supplement.

A Glossary of Useful Amino Acids
Amino acids are grouped together because they are often purchased from the same supplier; they can be bought in bulk and they tend to be much cheaper than other supplements.

Acetyl L-carnitine (ALCAR) is a naturally occurring amino acid produced in the body. Beef is the most abundant source of L-carnitine, which is a precursor to acetyl L-carnitine, though other red meats are also high in L-carnitine. Both acetyl L-carnitine and L-carnitine have similar properties, though acetyl L-carnitine can be taken on an empty stomach.

Acetyl L-carnitine and alpha-lipoic acid work synergistically and are often taken together with biotin (vitamin B7). A study at the Linus Pauling Institute in 2009 concluded that supplementing carnitine with alpha-lipoic acid improves memory, metabolism and energy levels. It also reported that taking these supplements as an adult decreases age-related damage to a variety of tissues such as brain tissues, skeletal muscle and the heart.

Acetyl L-carnitine is considered a nootropic. It turns body fat into energy and is important for muscle movement, cardiac function and many other functions. Because acetyl L-carnitine levels tend to reduce as we age, supplementation with this amino acid is likely to help with almost any degenerative disease. It has applications for a whole host of conditions, including:
• Alzheimer's disease, brain function and age-related memory loss
• Anti-aging
• Athletic performance and endurance
• Body-fat distribution and lypodystrophy
• Cataracts
• Chronic fatigue syndrome
• Down syndrome
• Facial paralysis
• Hair growth
• Nerve pain due to diabetes
• Peyronie's disease

If you wish to supplement with acetyl L-carnitine, 250 to 500 mg in the morning on an empty stomach is the usual recommended dose. Some people can tolerate higher doses, up to 1000 mg per day, without side effects.

A too high dose of ALCAR can interfere with sleep patterns, especially if taken at night; it can lead to agitation, an accelerated heartbeat and a feeling of nausea. If you experience any of these symptoms, reduce your dose accordingly. Because of ALCAR's propensity to burn fat, it can cause bad breath.

If you supplement with ALCAR, it is advisable to also supplement with biotin (vitamin B7) given that ALCAR, like ALA, depletes this vitamin, especially if ALCAR and ALA are taken together. Symptoms of biotin deficiency include hair loss etc.

Alpha-lipoic acid (ALA) is found naturally in meats (especially liver) vegetables and yeast. It is a most powerful antioxidant with many therapeutic uses. It helps mobilize body fat and metabolize sugars. It helps recycle other antioxidants: glutathione, vitamin E, vitamin C and coenzyme Q10.

Given its many anti-aging properties, alpha-lipoic acid is regarded by many as a veritable elixir. Alpha-lipoic acid is both fat and water-soluble and can counteract both fat-soluble and water-soluble free radicals in the organism. Supplementation with this amino acid can help with the following:
• Anti-aging
• Athletic endurance
• Cataracts, macular degeneration, diabetic retinopathy, glaucoma
• Chronic fatigue syndrome
• Detoxification
• Diabetes complications: blindness, nerve damage, reduces reliance on insulin
• Diminish the impact of chemotherapy on healthy tissue
• Heart disease
• Reduce the toxic side effects of the long-term use of medications, recreational drugs or anabolic steroids
• Multiple sclerosis if taken with vitamin D
• Post-workout recovery
• Regulates blood sugar, type 2 diabetes
• Represses HIV replication and infectivity
• Weight loss

As a supplement, ALA is usually taken in the more stable form, Na-Rala, in doses of between 50 to 500 mg a day. To help remove heavy metals dislodged by ALA from the body through the alimentary tract, include activated charcoal in your daily routine.

Given that ALA draws heavy metals out of tissues, people with high levels of mercury in their system may suffer adverse psychological reactions from a too high dose of ALA. Do not exceed 500 mg per day. Long term, it is advisable to have mercury fillings removed.

Many alpha-lipoic acid supplements on the market contain biotin (vitamin B7) in the formula. If not, it would be advisable to also supplement with biotin as ALA supplementation depletes this vitamin.

It is probably not advisable to supplement with such a powerful antioxidant continuously over a long period of time. If you have any medical condition or are taking any medication, especially insulin, always consult with your doctor before supplementing with ALA.

BCAAs are branch-chain amino acids: leucine, isoleucine and valine. These amino acids are considered essential in that they are not made by the body. They are found in most protein-rich foods. As supplements, they are usually mixed together.

BCAAs trigger protein synthesis and inhibits the breakdown of muscle. They improve glucose uptake and insulin sensitivity. BCAAs are noted for improving athletic performance. Supplementation with BCAAs can help with the following:
• Anorexia
• Brain function
• Endurance
• Bodybuilding
• Liver disease
• Muscle wasting
• Post-workout recovery
• Reduce visceral belly fat
• Type 2 diabetes

Though few people are likely to have a dietary deficiency of BCAAs, as they are contained in a huge variety of foods, supplementation provides a concentrated source that can be taken before workouts to improve performance and recovery. BCAA powder can be taken in 5g dosages 2 to 4 times a day. Because BCAA can lower blood-sugar levels, do not take as a supplement if you are taking insulin for type-1 diabetes.

Citrulline malate is a relatively new supplement on the market and considered by many bodybuilding pundits as the next big thing, though information regarding its benefits is relatively scarce. Citrulline malate is an amino acid that is a precursor to arginine and offers many of the same benefits, though is easier to digest, as it does not need to be taken on an empty stomach. Arginine stimulates the production of certain hormones, notably insulin and growth hormone, and is precursor to creatine.

Like arginine, citrulline malate increases nitric oxide production, which dilates blood vessels and facilitates blood circulation. It is also an anti-inflammatory. Citrulline malate is better than L-citrulline, a very similar

compound, at raising energy levels. Supplementing with citrulline malate can help with the following:
• Alzheimer's disease
• Athletic performance
• Bodybuilding
• Brain function and mental capacity
• Cardiovascular disease
• Congestive heart failure
• Erectile dysfunction
• Hypertension
• Immune function
• Kidney function
• Male infertility

Good quality citrulline malate should be in a 2:1 ratio. The usual recommended dose of citrulline malate is 4 to 8 grams per day, usually taken as a pre-workout an hour in advance. If you also supplement with L-arginine, reduce the supplementation of both amino acids accordingly. Always begin supplementation on a lower dose to adapt the digestive system lest you suffer stomach discomfort.

Creatine is an amino acid popular as a supplement with bodybuilders. It is synthesized in the body and found in small quantities in many protein-rich foods such as beef and fish.

Creatine increases IGF-1 (insulin-like growth factor) levels and ATP (adenosine triphosphate) which is used for energy. Creatine increases water retention in muscles, making them appear bigger. Supplementing with creatine can help with the following:
• Blood-glucose levels
• Brain function
• Endurance
• Protein synthesis
• Muscle size

Creatine is usually taken in 3 to 5 mg doses per day. Higher doses may have negative side effects such as dehydration or kidney damage. Though creatine can significantly increase muscle size, most of the increase dissipates once supplementation ceases.

In some people creatine can cause water retention if water consumption is not increased accordingly. There is also evidence that creatine supplementation can increase DHT levels, which can lead to hair loss in some, though this may be countered by supplementation with saw palmetto for those who are prone to hair loss.

HMB is a is synthesized in the body from protein in our food; it is a metabolite of the essential amino acid leucine, though it can also be found in small quantities in such foods as grapefruit, catfish and alfalfa.

HMB is an anti-catabolic agent useful for bodybuilders. It increases endurance by increasing VO2 max (maximal oxygen consumption). It also reduces metabolic acidosis. Supplementation with HMB can help with the following:
• Acidosis
• Aerobic performance
• Bodybuilding
• Body fat
• Endurance
• Hypertension and cardiovascular disease
• LDL cholesterol
• Recovery time
• Sleep apnea

HMB has no damaging side effects. It can be taken with other amino acids with anabolic properties such as arginine and glutamine.

The recommended dose is 3 grams a day for most individuals. For optimum results, this can be divided up into three 1-gram servings.

If you weigh more than 225 lbs, you can take up to 4 grams a day. If you weigh less than 125 lbs, 2 grams should suffice. It is not advisable that pregnant or lactating women take HMB.

L-arginine is an amino acid found in a wide variety of protein-rich foods. In the body, l-arginine converts into nitric oxide, which dilates blood vessels and facilitates blood circulation.

L-arginine is a precursor to creatine and stimulates the production of certain hormones, notably insulin and growth hormone. It is also an anti-inflammatory. Some of the benefits of supplementing with l-arginine include:
• Alzheimer's disease
• Athletic performance
• Bodybuilding
• Brain function and mental capacity
• Cardiovascular disease
• Congestive heart failure
• Erectile dysfunction
• Hypertension
• Immune function
• Kidney function
• Male infertility
• Type 2 diabetes

For the purpose of increasing HGH production, 5 to 9 grams of L-arginine are recommended per day. Always begin with a low dose of 2 to 3 grams per day and build up over two weeks to adapt the digestive system. Take half an hour to an hour before a workout on an empty stomach or before retiring to bed on an empty stomach.

If you have any health conditions for which you are taking medication, such as low blood pressure, a heart condition, diabetes, kidney problems or an active viral infection, always consult with your doctor before embarking on L-arginine supplementation.

L-glutamine is an amino acid produced in the body and is the most abundant amino acid in muscle tissue. It is a popular supplement with athletes, though it is much overlooked for its medicinal uses.

L-glutamine is an important supplement for intestinal cell health. It is an ideal supplement to give to anybody recovering from illness, cancer treatment or an operation. It is also considered a nootropic. Supplementing with L-glutamine can help with the following:
• Alleviate diverticulitis
• Anti-aging
• Bodybuilding
• Boosts t-cells and t-helper cells to bolster immune system
• Brain function
• Cell hydration
• Curbs cravings for sugary foods and alcohol
• Enhances nutrient absorption through intestines
• Gastrointestinal health
• Growth hormone synthesis
• Inhibit growth of some cancers
• Mood enhancer
• Post-workout recovery
• Prevents catabolic breakdown of muscle tissue when fasting or cutting
• Protein synthesis and positive nitrogen balance for muscle growth
• Repairs intestinal damage
• Weight gain for people with wasting diseases
• Weight/fat loss for dieters

Supplementation is usually in the region of 5 to 15 grams per day in divided doses. For the purpose of bodybuilding, supplementation of L-glutamine works best for older or unfit people. The effect on young, athletic types is likely to be negligible, though L-glutamine can be utilized for cutting in a low-calorie diet. There are no known negative side effects, though it is always advisable to begin on a lower dosage and build up over time.

L-leucine is an amino acid supplement popular with bodybuilders. It is found naturally in a variety of protein-rich foods such as meat and eggs.

L-leucine stimulates muscle synthesis, improves insulin sensitivity, regulates blood sugar and lowers cholesterol. L-leucine triggers an insulin spike in the absence of carbohydrates, thus lowering blood-sugar levels. Supplementation with L-leucine can help with the following:
• Bodybuilding
• Cholesterol
• Muscle protein synthesis
• Weight loss

The usual dose rage is between 2 and 5 grams taken with a protein shake. Do not take L-leucine in the evening lest you suffer a hypoglycemic episode during your nighttime fast. L-leucine will cause an insulin spike and should not be taken in a fasted state or if you are on a ketogenic diet.

An excessive intake of L-leucine can cause hypoglycemia even in the presence of carbohydrates in a meal. Do not take L-leucine if you suffer from hypoglycemia or are taking insulin for type-1 diabetes.

L-taurine is a non-essential amino acid that can be produced in the body and can be found in meat, fish and dairy products. However, it is not unusual to be deficient in taurine, especially as we age.

Taurine is a potent antioxidant and anti-inflammatory and plays an important role in many bodily functions. It elevates energy production and helps burn body fat, but unlike caffeine, it is a mild sedative and lowers cortisol levels. It dilates blood vessels, improves blood flow and increases oxygen supply to the brain and muscles. It improves insulin sensitivity.

L-taurine is often added to commercial energy drinks in relatively small doses. Supplementation with L-taurine can reverse many degenerative conditions associated with old age, and can help with the following:
• Accelerated recovery
• Alzheimer's disease and brain function
• Anti-aging
• Anxiety and stress
• Athletic performance and stamina
• Autoimmune diseases
• Blood pressure
• Cardiovascular health
• Cholesterol
• Hair growth
• Erectile dysfunction
• Liver function
• Testosterone

• Type-2 diabetes
• Vision
• Weight loss

The usual recommended dose of L-taurine is 2000 mg up to 3 times per day. L-taurine is well tolerated by the body with few notable side effects except in very large doses.

N-acetyl cysteine (NAC) is an amino acid and precursor to the powerful antioxidant glutathione. NAC is most noted for detoxifying the liver, as well as its many other remarkable rejuvenating properties. It is also considered a nootropic.

NAC is a relatively cheap supplement to buy and best taken with vitamin C in a ratio of 1:2. Supplementation with NAC can help with the following:
• Accidental poisoning
• Allergic rhinitis
• Alzheimer's disease
• Autoimmune diseases
• Angina
• Anti-aging
• Brain function
• Cancer
• Cardiovascular health and stroke
• Cirrhosis of the liver
• Chronic fatigue syndrome
• Detoxification
• Digestive problems
• Ear infections
• Elevated cholesterol
• Epilepsy
• Hay fever
• HIV
• Immune function
• Insulin sensitivity
• Liver and kidney health
• Multi-organ failure
• Radiation treatment
• Recovery from sports injuries
• Respiratory function

The recommended daily dose of NAC is between 200 and 1000 mg taken with twice as much vitamin C to prevent adverse side effects.

N-acetyl L-tyrosine is a non-essential amino acid found in meat, fish, dairy and whole grains. L-tyrosine is considered a nootropic. It is a precursor to a variety of neurotransmitters important to mental health and mental performance. Supplementation with N-acetyl L-tyrosine can be helpful to the following:
• ADD
• ADHD
• Alcohol and cocaine withdrawal symptoms
• Alzheimer's disease
• Chronic fatigue syndrome
• Depression and stress
• Erectile dysfunction
• Heart disease and stroke
• Low sex drive
• Maintain alertness at times of sleep deprivation
• Narcolepsy
• Parkinson's disease
• PMS
• Schizophrenia
• Weight loss

The recommended daily dose of N-acetyl L-tyrosine is between 200-500 mg. It is best taken in the morning and not combined with acetyl L-carnitine within the same 6-hour time frame, as they tend to cancel each other out.

Phosphatidyl-serene is a fat-soluble amino acid derivative that is highly prevalent in the brain. It is an essential component of cell membranes and considered a powerful natural nootropic, as it is the best natural supplement for memory, focus and mood stabilization.

The highest concentration of phosphatidyl-serene can be found is soya lecithin. Otherwise, it is found in various meats to varying degrees. Supplementing with phosphatidyl-serene can help with a variety of health conditions, including:
• Adrenal fatigue
• ADHD
• Alzheimer's disease
• Anxiety and depression
• Brain function
• Cortisol control
• Increased endurance and athletic performance
• Multiple sclerosis
• Weight loss

Doses of 100 to 500mg per day are recommended, depending on age or severity of condition. It is always advisable to start with a low dosage and build up to a higher dosage over time. Phosphatidyl-serene works synergistically with Omega 3.

Other Useful Supplements:

Activated charcoal is not really a supplement because it does not add anything to the diet. What it does do very efficiently is to eliminate from the intestinal tract all manner of undesirables: toxins, heavy metals, viruses, fungi, bacteria and intestinal gas. In that regard, activated charcoal can be used for a variety of things, including:
• Accidental poisoning, food poisoning, alcohol poisoning or drug overdose
• Candida, yeast infection and Candida toxins
• Cold and flu treatment
• Detoxification and detox symptoms
• Diarrhea
• Gastrointestinal health
• Hangover
• Flatulence
• Food intolerances
• Multiple sclerosis (which is triggered by toxins)

Take one to two flat tablespoons in one to two pints of water up to twice a day. Activated charcoal can be constipating if it is not taken with large amounts of water.

Activated charcoal will reduce stomach acidity and hamper food digestion, which is why it is best taken on an empty stomach. Never take activated charcoal within six hours of taking any medication or any other supplement, as it may be neutralized.

Aloe vera has a remarkable number of bioactive components including enzymes, amino acids, vitamins, minerals, fatty acids etc. It can come either as a gel for topical use or as a juice, which has a somewhat bitter taste.

For aloe vera to serve a medicinal purpose, it needs to be consumed in large quantities, which to many is not an exciting prospect. However, its medicinal properties are remarkable and it is one of the few natural food supplements that can be used to help with quite serious illnesses.

Aloe vera has anti-viral, anti-bacterial and anti-fungal properties. It boosts blood oxygen levels and replenishes enzymes, minerals, vitamins and glyconutrients, as well as improving electrolyte balance. It alkalizes the body, helping to normalize body PH. It is an anti-inflammatory and it increases blood viscosity.

Trials with aloe vera have shown it to be effective in treating both cancer and AIDS, managing to reverse the severity of both conditions. Aloe vera can certainly be used as an adjunct to conventional treatment. The healing properties of aloe vera juice are many and can help with the following:
• Arthritis
• Autoimmune diseases
• Athletic endurance
• Brain function
• Candida
• Cholesterol
• Constipation
• Diabetes complications
• Diarrhea
• Digestive aid
• Flatulence
• Heal the intestines and lubricate the digestive tract
• Hemorrhoids
• Hypertension and cardiovascular disease
• Hypoglycemia
• Immune function
• Stabilize blood sugar and help with diabetes
• Protects the kidneys from disease and helps prevent kidney stones
• Ulcers

As a gel, aloe vera can be applied topically to hydrate and heal the skin and treat all manner of skin complaints such as: acne, eczema, insect bites, psoriasis, rashes, cold sores, scaring and sunburn. The gel can be used as a natural water-based lubricant with condoms instead of KY gel, and because of its anti-viral, anti-fungal and anti-bacterial properties, it can increase protection against sexually transmitted diseases, including HIV.

Excessive consumption of aloe vera may cause diarrhea, but otherwise there is no recommended dose. Many commercial products are processed, heat-treated and diluted and have fewer health properties as a result, so be careful of what you buy.

Ashwagandha is an Ayurvedic herb called Indian ginseng because of its many adaptogenic properties. Apart from its antioxidant properties, it improves insulin sensitivity, stabilizes blood-sugar, enhances stamina and is most effective at countering stress and anxiety.

Ashwagandha is used to help the thyroid and the adrenals and to strengthen the immune system after an illness. Supplementation with Ashwagandha can be used for the following:

- Adrenal fatigue
- Alzheimer's disease and brain function
- Anxiety and depression
- Cancer and cancer reoccurrence
- Cholesterol
- Colds and flu
- Diabetes
- Hypothyroidism and hyperthyroidism
- Stamina and endurance

The recommended dosage is 500mg of standardized extract up to twice a day or 1000mg of powdered ashwagandha up to twice a day. Some people may suffer an adverse reaction, such as vomiting, to ashwagandha supplementation, so it is always advisable to begin with a small dose.

Astaxanthin is an antioxidant extracted from marine algae noted for its reddish pigment. It is a powerful anti-inflammatory and by far the most powerful natural antioxidant. It also has powerful UV-blocking properties useful to sunbathers. Supplementing with astaxanthin can help with the following:
- Allergies and autoimmune diseases
- Alzheimer's disease
- Anti-aging
- Arthritic pain
- Athletic endurance
- Brain function
- Cancer prevention and reoccurrence
- Detoxification
- Diabetes and diabetes complications
- Hypertension and cardiovascular disease
- Immune function
- Multiple sclerosis
- Parkinson's disease
- Physical endurance
- Protection against sun damage
- Reproductive health
- Vision: cataracts, macular degeneration, diabetic retinopathy, glaucoma
- Weight loss

The recommended dose of astaxanthin is 4-12 mg per day. The long-term effects of using such a powerful antioxidant constantly over many years have not been established. To be on the safe side, supplementation with astaxanthin should be cycled as part of a program of detoxification.

Vitamin B3 (niacin) is a water-soluble vitamin found in many common foods including certain meats, organ meats, tuna, mushrooms, seeds etc. Vitamin B3 dilates blood vessels and improves circulation. It also stimulates growth hormone. The benefits of supplementing with vitamin B3 include:
• Acne
• ADHD
• Alzheimer's disease
• Anti-aging
• Arthritic pain
• Athletic performance
• Brain function and memory loss
• Bodybuilding
• Cardiovascular health
• Cholesterol normalization
• Depression
• Diabetes and balancing blood sugar
• Eye disorders and cataracts
• Erectile dysfunction
• Hair growth
• Insomnia
• Migraine headaches
• Motion sickness
• Natural alternative to statins
• Schizophrenia
• Skin inflammation and blistering
• Tinnitus
• Weight loss

Vitamin B3 is contained in many commercial pre-workout preparations. However, B3 works synergistically with other B vitamins and any good vitamin B complex supplement should contain adequate amounts of B3 for most people.

Up to 500 mg of vitamin B3 can be taken per day, though high doses should not be taken over long periods of time because it can be toxic to the liver. Too much B3 intake can have many negative side effects including: water retention, headache, dizziness, nausea, ulcers, palpitations, increased allergic sensitivity etc. Vitamin B3 supplementation may also interact with certain medications.

Vitamin B6 (pyridoxal) is a collective term for several similar compounds of which pyridoxal 5-phosphate is the most biologically active. It is a powerful anti-inflammatory and plays an important role in nerve function, metabolism, liver function, immune function, skin health, eye health and in boosting energy levels. B6 is abundant in many staple foods, though food-processing techniques can dramatically deplete B6 content.

Alcoholism, chronic diarrhea, laxative abuse, steroid abuse and certain medications can deplete B6. Certain genetic disorders may hamper absorption of B6. Also if you consume a high-protein diet, supplementation with vitamin B6 may prove helpful. Supplementing with B6 may help with the following:

• Alzheimer's disease
• Anemia
• Anxiety and depression
• Arthritis
• Asthma
• Autism and brain function (with magnesium)
• Athletic performance
• Burning feat (diabetic neuropathy)
• Cardiovascular disease and stroke
• Chronic fatigue
• High blood pressure
• High cholesterol
• Immune function
• Kidney stones (with magnesium)
• Migraine headaches
• Muscle aches and pains
• Numbness and tingling in fingers (carpal tunnel syndrome)
• PMS
• Skin diseases
• Sleep disorders
• Water retention (ascites/edema)

For many conditions, vitamin B6 works synergistically with magnesium. Because vitamin B6 is water soluble, over-dosing should not be a problem, though pyridoxal 5-phosphate, the most biologically active form of B6, can be toxic if taken in doses above 100 mg per day or if fortified with other forms of B6. Vitamin B6 can interact with many drugs, so always consult your medical practitioner if you are taking any medication.

Benfotiamine is a much overlooked vitamin that can play an important part in countering many degenerative diseases. Because it is fat-soluble, benfotiamine is an especially potent form of vitamin B1, which is noted for protecting nerve function.

Foods that contain benfotiamine include: garlic, shallots, onions and leeks. Benfotiamine can be helpul in treating a variety of conditions associated with nerve damage. It is a useful supplement to take if you suffer

from reactive hypoglycemia, as it counters the harmful effects of low-blood sugar. Supplementation with benfotiamine may help with the following:
• Alzheimer's disease
• Anti-aging
• Arthritis
• Back pain
• Chemotherapy complications
• Congestive heart failure
• Diabetes complications
• Edema
• Fibromyalgia
• Hypertension and cardiovascular disease
• Insulin resistance
• Multiple sclerosis
• Neuropathy
• Sciatica
• Sleep apnea
• Thyroid disease
• Vision impairment
• Weight loss

A daily dose of 300-600mg of benfotiamine is recommended taken over the course of the day in divided doses. It is also advisable to take a vitamin B complex supplement with benfotiamine.

Vitamin C is the most widely used supplement and for many good reasons. Vitamin C supplements often contain added citrus bioflavonoids for greater bioavailability. Otherwise, vitamin C can either come in the form of acetic acid or calcium ascorbate.

Vitamin C bolsters the immune system by producing hydrogen peroxide, which helps destroy by oxidation all manner of infection as well as cancer cells. Though hydrogen peroxide is a precursor to free radicals, vitamin C also has antioxidant properties that serve to mop up the free radicals produced by the destruction of infection.

Vitamin C is essential for the synthesis of collagen, which helps maintain the health of the skin for a wrinkle-free and youthful appearance. It has anti-viral, anti-fungal and antibiotic properties. Vitamin C supplementation can help with the following:
• Anti-aging
• Cancer prevention and reoccurrence
• Candida
• Cardiovascular disease, stroke
• Digestive health
• Eye disease

• Immune function
• Prenatal health problems

Most people do not receive enough vitamin C in their diet, and a supplement of 500 mg a day is recommended. The upper limit for specific ailments is 6,000 mg per day in divided doses of no more that 2000 mg.

There is no toxicity to very high doses of vitamin C, as it is water-soluble. Any excess vitamin C is flushed out of the system, though doses at one time above 2000 mg may cause diarrhea.

If vitamin C supplementation irritates the stomach, calcium ascorbate, otherwise known by its trade name, Ester-C, is gentler on the stomach. Calcium ascorbate is a buffered, non-acidic version of vitamin C; it is more effective than acetic acid because it is more easily absorbed by the body and has a longer retention in the cells. Calcium ascorbate also provides calcium, in which case you may also need to supplement with magnesium to prevent a calcium/magnesium imbalance.

Chromium is a trace mineral popular with dieters and bodybuilders. It helps metabolize carbohydrates and helps stabilize blood-sugar levels.

Some of the natural sources of chromium include: beer, brewer's yeast, cereals, coffee, oysters, peas, potatoes, processed meats, rye, tea, thyme, whole-meal bread etc. A chromium deficiency is rare, but supplementation can help with the following:
• Alzheimer's disease and memory loss
• Cholesterol
• Cardiovascular disease
• Food cravings
• Hypertension
• Hypoglycemia
• Type 2 diabetes
• Weight loss

Dosage depends on type: chromium chloride 50 to 600mcg; chromium nicotinate 200 to 800mcg; chromium picolinate 300 to 1000mcg. Do not exceed the recommended dose.

Cordyceps is a type of mushroom used as a supplement to increase athletic performance. It increases lung capacity to provide more oxygen to the blood.

Cordyceps is the most effective supplement for increasing VO2. Other supplements that increase VO2 include: rhodiola rosea, HMB and iron. Supplementation with cordyceps can help with the following:
• Anti-aging
• Athletic performance

- Blood circulation
- Blood-glucose management
- Blood pressure
- Body building
- Brain function
- Cancer prevention/reoccurrence
- Chronic fatigue
- Erectile dysfunction and impotence
- High cholesterol
- Immune function
- Kidney function
- Respiratory illnesses
- Sleep apnea

The usual recommended dose is between 500 and 1000 mg per day. Cordyceps can lower blood-sugar levels and should not be taken if you are hypoglycemic, fasting, on a low-carbohydrate diet, or are taking insulin for diabetes. Nor should it be taken with other blood-sugar lowering supplements, such as leucine. Cordyceps is also a blood thinner and should not be taken before or after any surgical procedure.

Vitamin D3 can be synthesized in the body by simply exposing oneself to sunlight. However more people are deficient in vitamin D than any other vitamin for a variety of reasons, including the fact that certain chemicals can block the absorption of vitamin D, and certain medications can deplete vitamin D.

Supplementation with vitamin D3 is one of the simplest of solutions to a whole variety of health problems. The health benefits of vitamin D3 are numerous and include:
- Autoimmune diseases
- Bodybuilding
- Candida or bacterial overgrowth
- Cardiovascular health
- Depression and anxiety
- DNA repair
- Hormone imbalance
- Immune function
- Metabolic processes
- Strengthen teeth and bones
- Weight loss

For most adults, 2000-5000 iu per day of vitamin D3 is recommended. As a fat-soluble vitamin, vitamin D3 is best taken with oily food or a supplement such as Omega 3. Larger doses of vitamin D3 should always be taken with vitamin K2 to avoid any adverse side effects.

Dandelion root is known as the European ginseng and is widely recognized as an overall body tonic, detoxifier and a liver tonic that can help with jaundice. It aids in the proper flow of bile and stimulates the production of insulin.

Dandelion root is an appetite stimulator, digestive tonic, laxative and diuretic, and has remarkable anti-cancer properties. Supplementation with dandelion root extract can help with the following:
• Aching joints
• Anemia
• Appetite loss
• Bladder and kidney purification
• Bloating/intestinal gas
• Blood circulation
• Blood purification
• Blood sugar regulation
• Cancer prevention and reoccurrence
• Candida
• Cholesterol
• Congestion of the liver
• Constipation
• Detoxification
• Diabetes
• Digestion
• Fluid retention
• Gallstones
• Hypertension and cardiovascular disease
• Jaundice
• Muscle aches
• Skin infections
• Urinary tract infections
• Weight loss

As a supplement, choose the stronger dandelion-root extract rather than a product made from dandelion-root powder. Doses rage between 500 to 1000 mg per day. Dandelion root can also be eaten or prepared as a tea.

It is not advisable to take dandelion root if you are taking blood-sugar modulators, as this may give rise to hypoglycemia. Some people suffer an allergic reaction to dandelion root.

Vitamin E is a fat-soluble vitamin that can be found in a variety of foods, hence vitamin E deficiency is rare. Nevertheless, vitamin E is a popular supplement due to its strong anti-oxidant and anti-inflammatory properties, as well as its medicinal applications. Supplementing with vitamin E can help with the following:
• Anti-aging
• Allergies and autoimmune diseases
• Alzheimer's disease
• Arthritis
• Cataracts and age-related macular degeneration
• Diabetes and its complications
• Epilepsy
• Menopausal syndrome
• Night cramps
• Parkinson's disease
• PMS
• Restless leg syndrome

Daly doses can rage between 200 IU and 2000 IU. To take a higher dose, increase the dosage incrementally over two to three weeks so as not to shock the body, especially if you are elderly or have high blood pressure or heart disease.

Higher doses should not be contemplated for long-term use. Stay on a high dose for no more than a few weeks and then reduce the dosage incrementally over two to three weeks.

Always buy a natural rather than a synthetic vitamin E. Unfortunately most vitamin E supplements on the market are the synthetic variety called dl-alpha tocopheryl rather than the natural vitamin E called d-alpha tocopherol. Always read the label.

Used topically, vitamin E can rejuvenate skin and hair and reduce the appearance of wrinkles and scarring. It can be used as a nighttime moisturizer.

Evening Primrose Oil is high in gamma linolenic acid (GLA) and is a popular supplement with women, but can also be used by men. Many women use evening primrose oil to treat the symptoms of menopause.

Evening primrose oil had anti-inflammatory properties. The high gamma linolenic acid content can help prevent stretch marks and will give dull, aging skin a youthful glow.

Applied topically, it can be used to emolliate and hydrate the skin and treat skin complaints directly. Supplementation with evening primrose oil can help with the following:
• Acne
• Anti-aging

• Arthritis
• Menopause symptoms
• Skin conditions such as eczema and psoriasis
• Stretch mark prevention

In combination with gelatin and omega 3, supplementation with evening primrose oil should show a significant improvement in aging skin in just a few weeks. Most brands of evening primrose oil contain vitamin E to prevent oxidation. Doses of evening primrose oil can rage from 400 mg per day to 2000 mg per day.

Echinacea is an herb commonly used for colds and flu, but it has many other applications. Echinacea contains powerful immune-system stimulators and is an anti-inflammatory. It supports lymphatic function and strengthens macrophages, which are cells in the lymphnodes that excrete toxic waste from the lymph. The benefits of supplementing with Echinacea include:
• ADHD
• Anxiety and depression
• Arthritis
• Asthma
• Cancer and cancer reoccurrence
• Colds and flu
• Constipation
• Headaches
• Immune function
• Lymphedema
• Pain relief
• Skin conditions such as eczema and psoriasis

The recommended dose is 300 mg extract up to three times per day. Many commercial products that claim to contain Echinacea have been found to have no medicinal value whatsoever. Unless bought from a reputable company, it is best to buy the unadulterated herb and use it to make a tea with ½ to 1 g dried root.

Ginseng is another popular supplement with athletes. There are three forms of ginseng – Siberian, pannax and American – of which Siberian is arguably the most potent. All three types of ginseng are regarded as adaptogens, having the ability to normalize physiological functioning, strengthen the immune system, increase blood oxygen, strengthen the body and increase the body's ability to withstand the damaging effects of physical and emotional stress.

Ginseng can be used as an aphrodisiac for both men and women. All forms of ginseng increase the sperm count in men, though Siberian Ginseng is known to increase male testosterone levels.

Not only is ginseng considered a panacea, in that it can be used to help almost any ailment, healthy individuals can use it for increased strength, stamina and intelligence. As a stimulant, ginseng is best taken in the morning, though it may help with certain sleep conditions, such as obstructive sleep apnea. The health benefits of ginseng are many and may be used for the following:

• Aphrodisiac
• Alzheimer's disease
• Athletic performance
• Chronic fatigue syndrome
• Erectile dysfunction
• Immune function
• Memory and cognitive function
• Sleep apnea

Always begin with the recommended dosage when starting a course of ginseng and then gradually increase it if your body can tolerate it. If your dose is too high, it can cause headaches, insomnia, high blood pressure, nervousness and an irregular heart rate.

It is not advisable to supplement with any form of ginseng long term. Take occasional monthly breaks from supplementation and alternate between different types of ginseng. All forms of ginseng are not recommended for pregnant or lactating women.

Gingko biloba is an herbal supplement that dilates blood vessels and improves circulation, improving blood flow to the brain and enhancing memory function. It is considered a natural nootropic.

Gingko biloba acts as an anti-oxidant and inhibits the conversion of cholesterol into plaque. Gingko biloba can be used to help many conditions, including:

• Alzheimer's disease
• Erectile dysfunction
• Eye problems as a result of macular degeneration or diabetes
• Hemorrhoids
• Glaucoma
• Premenstrual syndrome
• Peripheral artery disease
• Raynaud's disease
• Vertigo
• Tinnitus (ringing in the ears)

Dosages for gingko biloba can vary between 40 mg a day to 360 mg a day in divided doses. A too high dose of gingko biloba can lead to: headache, dizziness, stomach upset, allergic skin reaction or pounding heartbeat. If any of these side effects are a problem, cut down on your dosage accordingly.

5-HTP is an extract from the seedpods of griffonia simplicifolia. It acts as a precursor to the neurotransmitter, serotonin, which performs many important regulatory functions.

Serotonin production declines with age and can be further depleted by many things, such as: stress, anxiety, sleep apnea, adrenal fatigue etc. Supplementing with 5-HTP can be used to help with many things, including:
• Adrenal fatigue
• Anxiety and depression
• Fibromyalgia
• Insomnia
• Migraines and chronic headaches
• PMS
• Weight loss

5-HTP has been shown to have significantly fewer side effects than prescription anti-depressants. However, doses higher than 400 mg may cause a headache.

For increased effectiveness, 5-HTP can be supplemented with other natural anti-depressants, such as: ashwagandha, benfotiamine, vitamin B complex, ginseng (all types), licorice root, N-acetyl L-tyrosine, phosphatidyl-serine, rhodiola, St. John's wart, valerian etc.

Iodine is a trace mineral and an essential component of thyroid hormone production. Iodine deficiency is believed to affect over 70% of the world's population.

Iodine controls metabolic rate and elevates energy levels. It helps detoxify the body of heavy metals, such as mercury, and can help prevent many types of cancer. Because iodine plays such an important role in hormone production, a severe deficiency can give rise to a myriad of ailments.

Foods rich in iodine include: seaweed, cod, cranberries, yoghurt, baked potato, raw milk, eggs. Supplementation with iodine may help with the following:
• Atherosclerosis
• Brain function and memory
• Breast cancer
• Constipation
• Cold hands and feet

- Cretinism
- Depression
- Dry skin
- Endemic goiter
- Fertility
- Fatigue
- Fibrocystic breast disease
- Headaches
- Hyperlipidemia
- Immune function
- Kidney function
- Menstrual problems
- Muscle weakness and joint stiffness
- Shortness of breath
- Thinning hair
- Weight loss

The recommended adult dosage of iodine is 290 mcg per day. Kelp supplements are high in iodine and also contain many other trace minerals.

Magnesium is one of the few minerals that a majority of people can supplement without the fear of putting other minerals out of balance. Magnesium needs to be in balance with calcium, but because most diets are abundant in calcium from dairy products, most people are deficient in magnesium. Withal stress and strenuous exercise can deplete the body of magnesium.

Magnesium is an anti-inflammatory and muscle relaxant. It plays an important role in metabolism and in brain function. Supplementation with magnesium is important to most age-related diseases. Supplementation can help with the following:
- Anxiety and depression
- Alzheimer's disease
- Arthritis
- Asthma
- Autism and ADD
- Collagen production
- Diabetes
- Fibromyalgia
- Fluid retention
- Hypertension and cardiovascular disease
- Inflammatory bowel disease
- Insomnia
- Impotence
- Lethargy

- Migraine headaches
- Muscle spasms and cramps
- Osteoporosis
- Restless leg syndrome
- Skin conditions
- Tooth cavities
- Urinary problems

The recommended base-line supplement is 5 mg per pound in body weight. Hence a 200 lb person would require 1000 mg per day. A higher dose may be taken if you are under stress or engage in regular strenuous exercise.

MCT oil is a medium-chain triglyceride usually derived from coconut oil. MCT oils include: caproic acid (C6), caprylic acid (C8), capric acid (C10) and lauric acid (C12). Caprylic acid and capric acid form the basis of most commercial MCT-oil products.

MCTs are easily digested to provide ketones as a source of energy, notably to the brain, without being stored as body fat. They are appetite suppressants and speed the metabolism. Like coconut oil, MCT oil is noted for its anti-fungal, antiviral and antibacterial properties. Supplementing with any MCT oil can help with the following:
- Alzheimer's disease and mental performance
- Candida overgrowth
- Chylous ascites
- Diabetes
- Endurance
- Hypoglycemia and blood sugar levels
- Insulin resistance
- Parkinson's disease
- Testosterone booster
- Viral infections
- Weight-loss

It is always advisable to introduce MCT oil slowly to the diet, as it can cause diarrhea and gastrointestinal problems. Caprylic acid is particularly useful in the treatment of Candida and Alzheimer's dementia.

MSM (methylsulfonylmethane) is an organic sulfur-containing compound that occurs naturally in a variety of foods but is easily destroyed by processing or over cooking. MSM stimulates collagen production and is a component of healthy bodily tissue. It is a powerful anti-inflammatory, antioxidant and calmative. It plays an important role in the production of glutathione, the master antioxidant, and can also bolster immune function.

MSM is called a miracle supplement for its many health benefits. It is also cheap to buy. Supplementation with MSM can help with the following:
• Allergies
• Alzheimer's disease and brain function
• Anti-aging
• Arthritis
• Asthma
• Cancer treatment and reoccurrence
• Circulation
• Constipation
• Detoxification
• Digestive problems and leaky gut syndrome
• Eye inflammation
• Fatigue
• Fibromyalgia
• Hair and nail growth
• Headache
• High blood pressure
• Joint pain and injury recovery
• Muscle pain and spasms
• Oral infections
• PMS
• Stamina
• Stress
• Stretch marks and scar formation
• Yeast infections

Used topically, MSM gel can be used for skin rejuvenation, hemorrhoids or to help with various aches and pains. Orally, MSM is best consumed in powder form mixed with water. Take 500 mg up to 3 times per day as a starting dose.

Some people may suffer bloating, in which case the starting dose can be reduced and taken on an empty stomach. Over time, the dosage maybe increased to up to 6 grams per day.

Nattokinase is a proteolytic enzyme extracted from natto, which is a fermented soy-based food. Nattokinase improves blood viscosity and is a powerful anti-inflammatory. It is also high in vitamin K2.

Nattokinase breaks down plaque build up in the arteries, including the brain, and lowers fibrin levels. It breaks down toxins and cellular debris in the blood and lymphatic system and undigested proteins in the gut. Supplementation with nattokinase can help with the following:
• Angina
• Alzheimer's disease

- Arthritis
- Athletic performance
- Autoimmune diseases/allergies
- Blood clots
- Blood pressure
- Cardiovascular health
- Circulation and blood flow
- Erectile dysfunction
- Gastrointestinal health
- Hemorrhoids
- Lymphedema and lymphatic drainage
- Scar amelioration
- Stroke prevention
- Varicose veins

Nattokinase is a cheaper alternative to serrapeptase and has many similar properties, though it is not as powerful. There are no known contraindications, but it is not advisable to take nattokinase with prescription blood thinners except under medical supervision.

There is no official recommended dose, but 100 mg, taken three times per day, should produce results. Nattokinase, taken with pycnoginol, can be used to prevent deep vein thrombosis on long-haul flights.

Omega 3 is an essential fatty acid found in a variety of foods. Few people today are likely to get an adequate intake of Omega 3 fats from their diet. It used to be found in reasonable amounts in beef and eggs, but due to modern animal feed, this has greatly declined.

Omega 3 is most abundant in oily fish such as: salmon, tuna and herring. For an adequate omega 3 intake, two or more servings per week of oily fish are recommended.

Flaxseed oil is an alternative vegetable source for omega 3, but the body does not absorb it as readily as fish oil. Other sources of omega 3 include: krill oil (most highly absorbable), canola oil, soybean oil, walnuts, pistachio nuts, sesame seeds, pumpkin seeds, poppy seeds and kale.

A low level of Omega 3 in the diet is a risk factor for cardiovascular disease and strokes and has been associated with depression. Omega 3 is the most prevalent fat in the brain and is needed for proper brain function.

Omega 3 has anti-inflammatory properties, as well as many other health benefits. Supplementation with Omega 3 may help with the following:
- Arthritis
- Blood-glucose regulation
- Brain function
- Cancer prevention and reoccurrence
- Cardiovascular health/stroke

- Cholesterol
- Digestive disorders
- Depression
- Immunity
- Macular degeneration
- Muscle and joint pains
- Skin problems

There is no recommended dose of Omega 3 and no known contraindications. Supplement with up to 7000 mg of per day in divided doses.

Because of contaminants from pollution in the sea, pregnant women are advised not consume large amounts fish-oil supplements. Flaxseed oil supplements may be preferable for those concerned about contaminants.

Potassium is the third most abundant mineral in the body. A high-protein diet requires increased potassium and magnesium to boost the metabolism, which is especially important to bodybuilders.

Potassium is an electrolyte that works with sodium to perform many essential bodily functions. It enhances bone health, regulates neural function, boosts metabolism, improves the nervous system, stabilizes blood pressure, strengthens muscles etc.

A whole variety of foods contain potassium, including: almonds, bananas, coconut water, chic peas, figs, grains, oranges, pistachios, prunes, peaches, poultry, salmon, tomatoes, vegetables, whole milk etc. However, because potassium needs to be in balance with sodium, most people consume far too much sodium in their diet, creating a greater need for potassium.

Potassium depletion can also be caused by: alcoholism, eating disorders, laxative abuse, diarrhea, diuretics, excessive sweating, certain dietary supplements and medications etc. If you have a potassium deficiency, supplementation can help with:
- Anemia
- Anxiety and stress
- Bloating
- Bodybuilding
- Cognitive function
- Constipation
- Depression
- Diabetes
- Irritable bowel disease
- Fatigue
- Fluid retention
- Hypertension and cardiovascular disease
- Hypoglycemia
- Metabolic function

- Migraine headaches
- Muscle weakness
- Palpitations
- Weight loss

There is no recommended dosage for potassium, but as a short-term remedy in conjunction with an improved diet, the usual dose is in the rage of 100 to 500 mg per day. Alternatively take a teaspoon a day of cream of tartar, which is very high natural source of potassium.

PQQ or pyrroloquinoline quinone is a powerful antioxidant prevalent in small amounts in many foods associated with healthy eating. PQQ enhances the production of new mitochondria and increases cellular energy production. PQQ increases a protein called DJ-1 important to brain health and function.

PQQ is considered a natural nootropic and anti-inflammatory. Supplementing with PQQ can help with the following:
- Alzheimer's disease
- Anti-aging and skin elasticity
- Arthritis
- Brain damage caused by stoke or injury
- Cancer prevention and reoccurrence
- Cardiovascular health
- Cognitive function and memory
- Depression
- Diabetes and insulin resistance
- Fatigue
- Metabolic rate
- Mood and mental health
- Neuron protection and nerve repair
- Parkinson's disease
- Weight loss

PQQ is water soluble and therefore non-toxic in high doses. Supplementation is usually in the rage between 5 to 20 mg. Higher doses maybe too stimulating for some people and cause headaches.

Quercetin is a plant pigment and bioflavonoid. It is a key component of many super foods. It is an antioxidant with anti-inflammatory, anti-histamine, anti-viral and anti-microbial properties. Supplementation with quercetin may help with the following:
- Allergies
- Asthma
- Arthritis

- Athletic endurance
- Cancer prevention and reoccurrence
- Cataracts and eye disorders
- Cholesterol
- Chronic fatigue syndrome
- Circulation problems
- Cognitive impairment
- Gout
- Hypertension and cardiovascular disease
- Inflammation of the prostate, bladder and ovaries
- Insulin resistance
- Leaky gut
- Prostate infections
- Skin disorders
- Stomach ulcers
- Viral infections

Doses are usually in the rage of 500 to 1000 mg twice daily. There are no known side effects, as it is a compound found abundantly in a healthy diet.

Rhodiola rosea, like ginseng, is considered an adaptogen. As such, it has the ability to correct imbalances in the body caused by mental or physical stress. It is a powerful antioxidant, a stimulant and fat burner.

In a similar way to ginseng, rhodiola can by used by otherwise healthy people to enhance physical and mental performance. Supplementing with rhodiola can help with the following:
- Athletic performance
- Brain function
- Depression and mild anxiety
- Fatigue
- Symptoms of multiple sclerosis
- Symptoms of sleep apnea
- Weight loss

A daily dose of rhodiola can range from 200 to 500 mg of a standardized extract twice daily. A too high dose may give rise to a headache.

Saw palmetto is a popular supplement for men, but it can be used by both genders to boost reproductive hormones and treat disorders of the urinary tract. Saw palmetto inhibits the conversion of testosterone to dihydrotestosterone (DHT).

Saw palmetto can prevent and to some extent reverse male-pattern baldness. It can also be used to prevent or treat an enlarged prostate. For this

purpose it can be taken with the herbal supplements Hydrangea and Horsetail. Supplementation of Saw palmetto can be used for the following:
• Acne
• Depression
• Male-pattern baldness
• Prostate enlargement.

There are no side effects to saw palmetto when taken in normal doses. Doses of saw palmetto can range from 300 mg to 3000 mg daily, given that DHT levels vary greatly from person to person. A man that is hirsute with markedly thinning hair is likely to have higher levels of DHT than the norm and as such require a higher dosage of saw palmetto.

Though saw palmetto may increase sex drive and help with depression, high doses taken over a long period of time can reverse these benefits and bring about depression, a reduced libido and erectile dysfunction. If any of these side effects are a problem, stop taking the supplement and start taking it again at a later date at a reduced dosage.

Serrapeptase is a proteolytic enzymes known to have miraculous healing properties. Other proteolytic enzymes include: nattokinase, pepsin, bromelain and papain, though serrapeptase is the most medicinally effective.

If taken with food, serrapeptase will simply help digest the food, but if taken on an empty stomach, it has remarkable health benefits including improving lymphatic function, eliminating scar tissue and working as a powerful anti-inflammatory. Serrapeptase can also be used to combat cancer. Cancer tumors cloak themselves with fibrinogen so that they go undetected by the immune system. Serrapeptase breaks down fibrinogen and helps remove the body of cancerous growths in the body.

There are no dietary sources for serrapeptase, which is an enzyme derived from the silk worm. Supplementing with serrapeptase can help with the following:
• Alzheimer's disease
• Angina
• Anti-aging
• Asthma
• Autoimmune diseases/allergies
• Arthritis
• Athletic performance and stamina
• Back pain
• Blood viscosity and blood clots
• Bronchitis
• Cancer and cancer reoccurrence
• Cardiovascular disease
• Carpal tunnel syndrome

- Cataracts
- Cholesterol
- Crohn's disease
- Chronic fatigue syndrome
- Cystic fibrosis
- Fibromyalgia
- Immune function
- Inflammatory bowel disease and IBS
- Liver cirrhosis
- Lupus
- Lymphedema
- Migraines
- Multiple sclerosis
- Nerve damage
- Prostate disease
- Rhinitis
- Scar tissue elimination
- Sinusitis
- Skin conditions such as eczema and psoriasis
- Sports injuries
- Stretch mark reduction
- Varicose veins
- Weight loss

The recommended dose of serrapeptase is between 80,000 and 250,000 IU taken an empty stomach. It is not advisable to take a high dose for a long period of time. As proteolytic enzymes improve blood viscosity, it is not advisable to take serrapeptase with blood-thinning medication or before an operation. Otherwise there are very few contraindications in supplementing with proteolytic enzymes.

Because proteolytic enzymes are fragile, processing may destroy their efficacy. Be wary of buying a cheaper product that has no medicinal value.

Sida cordifolia is an herb that has been used medicinally for over 2,000 years. It is a mild stimulant and appetite suppressant that has proved popular with athletes and dieters alike, but unlike caffeine and many other stimulants, Sida cordifolia is not catabolic.

Sida cordifolia has been noted for its ability to increase muscle strength and endurance. It possesses adaptogenic properties that can help normalize cortisol and blood-glucose levels during periods of stress.

It contains blood-sugar lowering properties. It is an anti-inflammatory with analgesic properties and can be used to treat aching joints and bones, edema and headaches. It is a potent antioxidant and liver protector, especially from alcohol-induced toxicity.

It is rejuvenating to the nervous, circulatory and urinary systems. It is a decongestant useful in the treatment of colds and allergic rhinitis. It is a mild diuretic and diaphoretic. Supplementation may help with the following:
• Alzheimer's disease
• Arthritis
• Asthma
• Athletic endurance
• Brain function
• Bronchopulminary conditions
• Cold and flu
• Diabetes
• Headache
• Fatigue
• Fluid retention
• Rhinitis
• Weight loss

Sida cordifolia is used in a variety of weight-loss products. Supplements of Sida cordifolia usually come in doses of up to 350 mg to be taken once a day.

If you suffer from any of the following side effects, immediately desist from using Sida cordifolia, though you may wish to restart taking it at a later date at a lower dose: irritability, nervousness, rapid heartbeat, shortness of breath, headaches, dizziness, itching, elevated body temperature, vomiting. If symptoms are severe, it is advisable to seek the advice of a healthcare professional.

If you have any of the following conditions, it is not advisable to supplement with Sida cordifolia: heart disease, high blood pressure, type 1 diabetes, hypoglycemia, epilepsy, thyroid disease, angina, recurring headaches, bleeding disorder, glaucoma, enlarged prostate, a psychiatric condition. Sida cordifolia is not recommended for pregnant or lactating women.

Spirulina is best described as a food supplement; it is an algae and usually bought in either a powder or a capsule form. It is one of the most potent sources of nutrients: high in essential amino acids, essential fatty acids, antioxidants, B vitamins, notably B12, and minerals.

Its iron content is notable for being bio-available and will not cause constipation. It is also high in chlorophyll, which helps to detoxify the blood and boosts the immune system.

Spirulina can combine with heavy metals and remove them. It is also believed to help counteract the effects of exposure to radiation, notably chemotherapy.

Spirulina is approximately 65% protein, containing all of the essential amino acids. It is one of the few natural sources of the essential fatty acid, gamma linolenic acid, which is an anti-inflammatory. It also contains omega 3, 6 and 9.

Spirulina contains over 26 times as much calcium as milk. It is also high in vitamin D, making it an ideal supplement for those suffering from osteoporosis. Supplementation with spirulina may help with the following:
• Alzheimer's disease
• Anti-aging
• Arthritis
• Anemia
• Detoxification
• Osteoporosis
• Weight loss

Always chose an organic source of spirulina, as other sources may be contaminated with pollutants or additives. It may be consumed in capsule form, but a cheaper and more reliable source is in the form of an unadulterated powder, which may be added to a smoothie.

As a food supplement, there is no recommended dose for spirulina, but 2 teaspoons per day should suffice. During illness, 2 to 3 tablespoons per day are recommended.

Chlorella is an alternative to spirulina, but has a stronger taste that is not to everybody's liking. However, chlorella is noted for its remarkable detoxification properties, not least the elimination of heavy metals such as lead and mercury.

Triphala is a staple of Ayurvedic medicine and means *three fruits*. It is an herbal formulation high in flavonoids and polyphenols, which have antibacterial, anti-inflammatory and anti-diarrheal properties. Triphala is considered an overall tonic.

Triphala removes toxins from the intestinal tract and helps with the absorption of nutrients. It can be used as a laxative without the harmful side effects of commercial laxatives. For this reason, it is a useful supplement to take during a program of detoxification. Supplementation with triphala can help with the following:
• Arthritis
• Cancer and cancer reoccurrence
• Cholesterol
• Colon cleansing
• Constipation
• Multiple sclerosis
• Weight loss

The recommended dose of powdered triphala is 1 teaspoon on an empty stomach, preferably before bed. Start with ½ teaspoon for the first week or so lest you suffer any gastrointestinal problems. The detoxification of the digestive tract can cause increased intestinal gas. An excessive intake of triphala can cause diarrhea.

Wheatgrass is a popular food supplement because of its high nutritional content. It is the young grass of the common wheat plant and can be purchased in a variety of forms, including juice and powder.

Wheatgrass is packed with chlorophyll, vitamins, minerals and amino acids. It is an anti-inflammatory and can help oxygenate, alkalinize and detoxify the body. Supplementing with wheatgrass can help with the following:
• Allergies
• Alzheimer's disease
• Anemia and strengthening of blood
• Anti-aging
• Arthritis
• Blood-sugar regulation
• Brain function
• Cancer prevention and reoccurrence
• Digestion
• Endurance
• Fertility
• High cholesterol
• Immune function
• Liver function
• Multiple sclerosis
• Side effects of chemotherapy
• Skin complaints
• Sleep disorders
• Weight loss

Wheatgrass is a raw food and as such there is no recommended dosage. In powdered form, begin with a teaspoon per day for the first few weeks in order to build up a tolerance and build up to a tablespoon.

Zinc is a trace mineral important to immune function, the repair and functioning of DNA, metabolic functions including glucose metabolism, the nervous system, reproductive health and wound healing. Zinc is also an antioxidant and anti-inflammatory.

Food sources of zinc include: almonds, ginger root, meat, oats, oysters, peas, peanuts, pecans, pumpkin seeds, turnips, whole meal bread. Supplementation with zinc can help with the following:
• Alzheimer's disease and cognitive function

- Appetite loss
- Athletic performance and endurance
- Autoimmune diseases
- Cancer/cancer reoccurrence
- Cardiovascular health
- Depression
- Diabetes
- Eczema
- Fatigue
- Fertility in both men and women
- Hair loss/alopecia
- Immune function
- Insulin sensitivity
- Loss of taste and smell
- Low-blood pressure
- Night vision
- Prostate disorders
- Testosterone production
- Weight loss

People most susceptible to zinc deficiency include: alcoholics, vegetarians, people with eating disorders and people with digestive problems or low stomach acid, which is not so rare. The usual recommended daily dosage is 50mg per day.

Chapter Ten

The Dietary Index of Everyday Foods

For the purpose of planning meals for the purpose of food combining, it is important to know the dietary content of many everyday foods. Carbohydrate foods with the highest glycemic index tend to have the highest insulin response. Though protein produces a much lower insulin response than carbohydrate, a high protein content nevertheless gives rise to a higher insulin response than a low protein content. Furthermore, when carbohydrate foods and protein foods are combined in the same meal, the insulin response is accumulative, often giving rise to an insulin spike.

The Glycemic Index of Common Carbohydrate Foods

Low Glycemic Index Carbohydrates:
• Roasted and salted peanuts – 14
• Low-fat yoghurt with sweetener – 14
• Cherries - 22
• Grapefruit – 25
• Pearl barley – 25
• Red lentils – 26
• Whole milk – 27
• Dried Apricots – 31
• Butter beans – 31
• Fettucine pasta – 31
• Skimmed milk – 32
• Low-fat fruit yoghurt – 33
• Whole-wheat spaghetti – 37
• Apples – 38
• Pears – 38
• Tomato soup (canned) - 38
• Apple juice – 40
• Noodles – 40
• Spaghetti – 41
• All Bran – 42
• Chick peas – 42

- Peaches – 42
- Macaroni – 45
- Grapes (green) - 46
- Orange juice – 46

Moderate Glycemic Index Carbohydrates:
- Muesli – 56
- Boiled potatoes – 56
- Sultanas - 56
- White pitta bread – 57
- White rice – 58
- Honey – 58
- Margareta pizza – 60
- Ice cream – 62
- New potatoes – 63
- Coca cola – 63
- Raisins – 64
- Couscous – 65
- Rye bread – 65
- Pineapple – 65
- Cantaloupe melon – 67
- Croissant – 67
- Shredded wheat – 68
- Weetabix – 69
- Wholemeal bread – 69

High Glycemic Index Carbohydrates:
- Mashed potato - 70
- White bread – 70
- Watermelon – 72
- Swede – 72
- Bagel – 72
- French fries – 75
- Jelly beans – 80
- Rice cakes – 82
- Rice Krispies – 82
- Cornflakes – 84
- Jacket potato – 85
- Baguette – 95
- Parsnips – 97
- White rice, steamed – 98

Protein Content of Common Protein-Rich Foods
Dairy:
- 100 g of whey protein isolate provide 90 g of protein.

- 100 g of whey protein provide 80 g of protein.
- 100 g of unprocessed hard cheese provide 25 g of protein.
- 100 g of haloumi provide 21g of protein.
- 100 g of goat/sheep cheese provide 17 g of protein.
- 100 g of unprocessed cream cheese provide 11 g of protein.
- 100 g of ricotta provide 10 g of protein.
- 100 g of full-fat yoghurt provide 6 g of protein.
- 1 large egg provide 6 g of protein.
- 100 ml of cow's milk provide 4 g of protein.

Meat, Poultry and Fish:
- 100 g of skinless chicken breast provide 34 g of protein.
- 100 g of lamb/lamb chops provide 28 g of protein.
- 100 g of beef provide 27 g of protein.
- 100 g of snapper provide 27 g of protein.
- 100 g of tuna provide 26 g of protein.
- 100 g of salmon provide 22 g of protein.
- 100 g of turkey provide 22 g of protein.
- 100 g of bacon provide 22 g of protein.
- 100 g of ham provide 17 g of protein.
- 100 g pork sausage provide 17 g of protein.
- 100 g beef sausage provide 14 g of protein.

Nuts and Seeds:
- 100 g of peanuts provide 26 g of protein.
- 100 g of almonds provide 24 g of protein.
- 100 g of cashew nuts provide 20 g of protein.
- 100 g of walnuts provide 16 g of protein.
- 100 g of brazil nuts provides 13 g of protein.
- 100 g of sunflower seeds provide 27 g of protein.
- 100 g of pumpkin seeds provide 24 g of protein.

Legumes:
- 100 g of firm tofu provide 12 g of protein.
- 100 g of silky tofu provide 8 g of protein.
- 100 g of red lentils provide 7 g of protein.
- 100 g of yellow split peas provide 7 g of protein.
- 100 g of kidney beans provide 7 g of protein.
- 100 g of chickpeas (garbanzo) provide 6 g of protein.
- 100 g of cannelini beans provide 6 g of protein.
- 100 g of quinoa provide 4 g of protein.

Bread and Grains:
- 100 g of white bread (approx 2 slices) provide 10 g of protein.
- 100 g of gluten-free bread provide 10 g of protein.

- 100 g of whole-meal bread provide 9 g of protein.
- 100 g of rye bread provide bread 9 g of protein.
- 100 g of whole-meal pasta provide 5 g of protein.
- 100 g of white pasta provide 4 g of protein.
- 100 g of rice provide 3 g of protein.
- 100 g of pearled barley provide 3 g of protein.
- 100 g of polenta, cooked in water, provide 3 g of protein.
- 100 g of raw oats provide 2 g of protein.

A Message From the Author
Thank you for taking time to read this book. I hope it has given you many practical and useful tips in your quest for rejuvenation. Where there is a will and a vision, all things are possible.

If you found this book enlightening in any way, I would be very grateful if you post a short review on Amazon. As a self-published writer, your support can make a big difference.

You can follow me on twitter: @DooryLaith

Wishing you the best of health, happiness and success in all your pursuits.

All the best,
Laith